Outpatient Hip and Knee Replacement

R. Michael Meneghini • Leonard T. Buller
Editors

Outpatient Hip and Knee Replacement

Implementation and Essential Techniques

Springer

Editors
R. Michael Meneghini
Department of Orthopedic Surgery, Indiana
University School of Medicine
Indiana Joint Replacement Institute
Indianapolis, IN, USA

Leonard T. Buller
Department of Orthopedic Surgery
Indiana University Health
Fishers, IN, USA

ISBN 978-3-031-27036-9 ISBN 978-3-031-27037-6 (eBook)
https://doi.org/10.1007/978-3-031-27037-6

This Springer imprint is published by the registered company Springer Nature Switzerland AG
The registered company address is: Gewerbestrasse 11, 6330 Cham, Switzerland

Preface

We are in the midst of an outpatient revolution! Ten years ago, most orthopaedic surgeons and healthcare providers would not have dreamed that the majority of total hip and knee arthroplasty procedures would be performed in the outpatient setting discharged to home within hours of their surgeries. Accelerated by the COVID-19 global pandemic which constrained hospital beds and resources, we are on a trajectory to where the majority of patients undergoing primary total hip and knee arthroplasty are discharged to home the same day. However, due to the medical and surgical complexity of these procedures and patients who they are performed on, sophisticated programmes composed of high-functioning healthcare providers with highly coordinated care pathways and protocols must be developed and maintained.

This book provides real-world and practical content from nationally and internationally recognized experts in outpatient hip and knee arthroplasty. They share their insights on all the essential elements needed to develop a robust and successful outpatient same-day-discharge hip and knee arthroplasty program. All the critical issues are covered in the following text and include patient selection, perioperative medical optimization and management, perioperative pain control and anaesthetic techniques, common threats to patient discharge, patient connectivity and monitoring outside the hospital as well as financial considerations. The reader will find all the essential elements to develop and implement their own same day discharge outpatient hip and knee program in either a hospital or ambulatory surgery centre setting.

Indianapolis, IN, USA — R. Michael Meneghini
Fishers, IN, USA — Leonard T. Buller

Acknowledgements

To my amazing wife, Sarah. Sharing your life with an academic orthopaedic surgeon is challenging. Your immeasurable love, support, loyalty and selfless sacrifice is awe-inspiring. I am blessed and eternally grateful. To my six wonderful children, Ethan Angelo, Cecilia, Gianna, Luca, Mario and Milania. I am grateful for your love and support and so proud of the compassionate, empathetic and uniquely talented individuals you have all become. To my late mother, you are an inspiration in survival, love, passion, perseverance and true success in life. To my mentors, I am eternally grateful for your inspiration, education and encouragement. I truly "stand on the shoulders of giants". To my colleagues on this incredible journey transforming hip and knee arthroplasty to an outpatient procedure, in particular Dr. Pete Caccavallo, Dr. Mark Nielson and Dr. David Conrad. I am honoured and humbled by your partnership, collaboration and friendship and acknowledge this would not have been possible without you. Finally, to my colleague, friend and co-editor, Dr. Lenny Buller. Your expertise, dedication and partnership enabled this book to happen and I cannot thank you enough.

Contents

1 **Patient Selection for Same-day Discharge: Medical and Surgical Risk Assessment** 1
Peter Caccavallo and R. Michael Meneghini

2 **Medical Optimization and Risk Mitigation for Readmission** 9
Vignesh K. Alamanda and Bryan D. Springer

3 **Surgical Appropriateness for Outpatient TJA in an ASC** 17
Jesua Law, David A. Crawford, and Adolf V. Lombardi

4 **Essential Components of Preoperative Education and Planning** 25
Alexander Sah

5 **Multimodal Pain Management Protocols for THA and TKA** 37
Elizabeth B. Gausden, Mark W. Pagnano, and Matthew P. Abdel

6 **Surgical Techniques and Protocols to Minimize Blood Loss and Postoperative Pain** 49
Nathanael Heckmann and Scott Sporer

7 **Anesthesia for Outpatient TJA: Anesthetic Techniques and Regional Blocks** 59
Mark E. Nielson

8 **Threats to Same Day Discharge: Prevention and Management** 77
Charles P. Hannon, Parag D. Patel, and Craig J. Della Valle

9 **Is there an Optimal Place for Outpatient TJA: Hospital, ASC, or "Other"?** 85
William G. Hamilton, Roshan T. Melvani, and Agnes D. Cororaton

10 **Navigating the Limitations and Obstacles of TJA in a Free-Standing ASC** 91
Nicholas B. Frisch and Richard A. Berger

11 Same-Day Discharge in the Hospital: Resources and Program Elements . . . 105
Gregory G. Polkowski and Michael D. Gabbard

12 Discharge the Day of Surgery: Strategies to Optimize and Discharge Criteria . . . 113
Joshua C. Rozell, Dimitri E. Delagrammaticas, and Raymond H. Kim

13 Staying Connected with the Patient after Discharge: Strategies and Resources . . . 121
Tony S. Shen, Patawut Bovonratwet, and Michael P. Ast

14 Physical Therapy Following Same-Day Discharge Total Joint Arthroplasty . . . 127
Matthew J. Grosso and William Hozack

15 Strategies to Minimize Patient Anxiety, Emergency Room Visits, and Readmissions Following Outpatient Total Joint Arthroplasty . . . 135
Charles De Cook

16 Making the Transition to Outpatient: Resources and Pathway Changes . . . 147
Paul K. Edwards, Jeffrey B. Stambough, Simon C. Mears, and C. Lowry Barnes

17 Outcome Metrics: What to Measure Now and in the Future . . . 157
Robert Pivec and Jess H. Lonner

18 How to Mitigate Risk for Surgeons, Institutions, and Patients . . . 165
Leonard T. Buller and R. Michael Meneghini

19 Financial Considerations for Surgeons in the Outpatient Setting: Costs and Ownership Models . . . 177
Joe Zasa

20 Outpatient Hip and Knee Arthroplasty: Implications for Hospitals, ASCs, and Payers . . . 185
John R. Steele and Michael P. Bolognesi

Index . . . 191

Chapter 1
Patient Selection for Same-day Discharge: Medical and Surgical Risk Assessment

Peter Caccavallo and R. Michael Meneghini

Introduction

Total hip and knee arthroplasty (THA, TKA) performed in the outpatient setting has become increasingly utilized due to multiple factors and there are multiple studies that demonstrate efficacy for primaries [1, 2] and carefully selected revision cases [3–6]. The factors driving utilization of outpatient hip and knee arthroplasty surgeons include investment in ambulatory surgery centers (ASCs); repercussions of the COVID-19 pandemic such as constrained hospital resources and increased patient demand; and Centers for Medicare and Medicaid Services (CMS) decisions with the removal of these procedures from the inpatient-only list. Furthermore, case volume projections for primary THA and TKA being performed in ASCs are projected to increase by 457% and 633%, respectively over the next decade [7]. Nevertheless, as more arthroplasties are performed in the outpatient setting, thorough medical evaluation and proper patient selection and optimization will become more critical for safe and effective rapid discharge. This chapter will highlight key elements related to medical evaluation and patient selection and optimization for outpatient total joint replacement.

P. Caccavallo
Perioperative Medicine, Indiana Joint Replacement Institute, Indianapolis, IN, USA
e-mail: pcaccavallo@injri.com

R. M. Meneghini (✉)
Department of Orthopaedic Surgery, Indiana University School of Medicine, Indiana Joint Replacement Institute, Indianapolis, IN, USA
e-mail: mmeneghini@injri.com

R. M. Meneghini, L. T. Buller (eds.), *Outpatient Hip and Knee Replacement*,
https://doi.org/10.1007/978-3-031-27037-6_1

Medical Evaluation and Patient Selection

Many joint replacement surgeons limit their outpatient surgical practice to the healthiest of patients. However, the vast majority of patients with end-stage arthritis fail to fall into this category which greatly limits the number of patients eligible for outpatient surgery. The key to *outpatient* surgical selection is to identify the patient who will safely discharge on the same day and is at a low risk for readmission, especially within the first 2 days. This is different than just identifying those who have increased risk for a postoperative medical *complication* within 90 days of surgery, which is the basis for most risk calculators. For example, a patient with *stable* coronary artery disease who has reasonable exercise tolerance will be more likely to discharge the same day after a total hip or knee arthroplasty. On the contrary, a healthy patient with a history of poor postoperative pain tolerance would be a low medical risk, but a high risk of failure for same-day discharge due to poor pain control. Further, an otherwise healthy patient with a history of postoperative urinary retention would be problematic in terms of discharging the same day. Simply put, increased medical complication risk does not necessarily equal the risk of outpatient failure. There are many variables including psychological, social, and medical risks that will allow one to effectively screen for appropriate outpatient candidates.

There are many *medical* risk assessment tools available (i.e., ASA, CCI, RAPT) [8–10] but they were never intended to be used as an outpatient screening tool. The most common classification system is the American Society of Anesthesiologists (ASA) Physical Status Classification originally described in 1976 [8]. The ASA score is based on a survey of 255 anesthesiologists used to determine the health status of a patient based on a 1–5 scale. A score of 1 represents a "normal healthy patient," 5 indicates a patient that is about to die, and 4 is a patient with a medical condition that is "a constant threat to life." This leaves most patients with a score of 1, 2, or 3 for elective TJA. Separating patients into three categories is a poor screening tool for outpatient surgical selection as the score is not particularly discerning. The authors of the original ASA publication even admit the classification system "suffers from a lack of scientific precision" [8].

Furthermore, all patients should undergo a complete history and physical medical exam for identification of modifiable risk factors as well as appropriateness for elective surgery from a cardiac standpoint using the most recent American College of Cardiology and American Heart Association guidelines. Laboratory and cardiac testing should be obtained for all patients based on current perioperative guidelines including hemoglobin, creatinine, and HgA1c values. A physical exam is performed with special attention to cardiac, pulmonary, and neurological baseline abnormalities that delineate a clear physical baseline and avoidance of postoperative misunderstandings. In our outpatient program, patients are stratified using the Outpatient Arthroplasty Risk Assessment (OARA) Score [11] which consists of nine categories including General, Hematological, Cardiac, Endocrine, Gastrointestinal, Neurological/Psychological, Renal/Urology, Pulmonary, and Infectious disease. The OARA Score has demonstrated near-perfect positive predictive values (PPV) of

91.5 and 98.8; and very low false positive rate values of 3.0 and 0.7 using cut-off values of 59 and 79, respectively for determining which arthroplasty patients are safe for early discharge in the outpatient setting [11, 12]. This score has also been externally validated outside the original institution with a PPV of 86.1 for both same-day and next-day discharge of THA patients in a rapid discharge program [13]. The OARA Score, compared to other *medical* risk stratification tools, provides a higher level of scientific precision as the score ranges from 0 to 100 on a continuous scale compared to the ASA classification ranging from 1 to 5 on a categorical scale. It is also important to note the OARA Score was not designed to be a measure of physical status, medical complexity, or mortality. Key aspects of the OARA Score are briefly summarized below:

General Medical

A patient's general overall health and functional status are assessed. It is intuitive that a patient with no home support and severe deconditioning is a poor outpatient candidate. Obesity and morbid obesity, while not prohibitive to outpatient surgery, tend to predict patients with poorer states of health and decreased medical compliance. Screening for high narcotic and benzodiazepine tolerance or simply a history of chronic pain control difficulties are barriers to physical and mental readiness for same-day discharge. The General Medical category accounts for 180 possible points contributing to the overall original OARA Score.

Hematological

Patients with anemia, especially significant or unevaluated anemia, can potentially have a wide variety of known and unknown medical problems which can be exacerbated in the immediate postoperative period. With large expected blood loss, patients with likely postoperative transfusion necessity should be avoided. Those with difficulty managing anticoagulation/antiplatelet medications will require more attention and sometimes increase the risk of outpatient failure. The Hematological category accounts for 325 possible points contributing to the overall original OARA Score.

Cardiac

While patients with stable coronary artery disease can make great outpatient candidates, identifying those with tenuous conditions despite appropriate management can be a challenge. With large fluid shifts, as well as intentional and unintentional intraoperative hypotension, this may exclude patients with severe aortic stenosis or a history of pulmonary edema. These patients frequently require longer periods of postoperative monitoring as an inpatient. The Cardiac category accounts for 385 possible points contributing to the overall original OARA Score.

Endocrine

Uncontrolled diabetes is not only a marker for perioperative complications but also noncompliance. Outpatient surgery requires increased responsibility on the side of the patient. Those that show poor long-term compliance often will show poor short-term compliance and an increased risk of readmission. Adrenal suppression can make the aforementioned expected hypotension difficult to manage within the first 24 h. The Endocrine category accounts for 165 possible points contributing to the overall original OARA Score.

Gastrointestinal

Patients with cirrhosis are high-risk patients in general. However, healthy patients with a history of postoperative ileus and difficulty swallowing can be at high risk for postoperative complications and readmissions. The Gastrointestinal category accounts for 185 possible points contributing to the overall original OARA Score.

Neurological/Psychological

Patients with dementia are a challenge, even on the inpatient side. Postoperative rehabilitation, expected pain, and detailed medicine directions can be quite intimidating. It is often unpredictable who will tolerate anesthesia and postoperative sedating medications or who will have prolonged postoperative delirium. Even patients suffering from depression alone can find simple instructions challenging to follow and are better treated as inpatients. The Neurological/Psychological category accounts for 185 possible points contributing to the overall original OARA Score.

Renal/Urology

Chronic renal disease is also very sensitive to fluid shifts and hypotension and frequently will require specific fluid and medicinal adjustments beyond the day of surgery. With a significant incidence of anesthetic-induced postoperative urinary retention (POUR), patients with a history of POUR, or uncontrolled benign prostatic hyperplasia (BPH) can be a challenge unless protocols are in place to manage this common issue. The Renal/Urology category accounts for 220 possible points contributing to the overall original OARA Score.

Pulmonary

Patient with tenuous asthma or chronic obstructive pulmonary disease (COPD) need special consideration of its predicted stability postoperatively. Untreated sleep apnea can be especially dangerous when postoperative pain and narcotic requirement are at their peak on postoperative day zero. The Pulmonary category accounts for 250 possible points contributing to the overall original OARA Score.

Infectious Disease

The overall stress and physical demand for joint replacement is significant. Patients with significant acute infections regardless of potential prosthetic joint infection risk are a risk for same-day discharge failure. The Infectious Disease category accounts for 65 possible points contributing to the overall original OARA Score.

In addition to a medical risk stratification tool, program, or methodology such as OARA, appropriate medical evaluation should include thorough medical history and physical examination directed toward the psychological, social, and medical issues that will predict the likelihood of outpatient safety and success. It is sometimes difficult to determine if a *medical* risk factor confers a higher likelihood of delay in outpatient discharge. An appropriate medical evaluation that includes a validated tool to identify risks for outpatient failure will open outpatient surgery to a much larger population of patients that may have increased medical risks but would still be appropriate for outpatient surgery. It not only provides patient assurance and a guide for appropriate screening, but it provides an appropriate defense for unforeseen and unavoidable complications that still rarely occur in all settings.

Perioperative Optimization

In addition to patient selection, perioperative patient optimization is also critical to successful early discharge of outpatient arthroplasty patients. This involves multidisciplinary perioperative protocols developed in conjunction with anesthesia and a dedicated internal medicine specialist [14]. Protocols prioritize intraoperative fluid management and resuscitation, multimodal pain control, and overall consistent surgical care (i.e., approach and operative time). Intraoperative fluid management should emphasize euvolemia via protocols designed to allow/encourage patients to drink clear liquids up to 2 h before surgery. We emphasize euvolemia rather than hypovolemia or overhydration with excessive fluid loading, both of which can exacerbate postoperative urinary retention. Then, approximately 2 L of fluid is given intraoperatively to maintain adequate tissue perfusion and oxygen delivery [15]. Pain control protocols should highlight multimodal medications given preoperatively and postoperatively [16]. Intraoperative pain control can be managed effectively with nerve blocks and peri-articular injections, particularly for knees [17, 18]. Further, protocols should prioritize conserving intraoperative blood loss with the use of tranexamic acid (TXA) [19, 20] and potentially advanced technology such as abbreviated navigation of the femur which has shown to reduce blood loss during joint replacement [21]. Postoperatively, an extended antibiotic prophylaxis protocol has shown to reduce infection rates associated with primary and revision TJA [22–24]. While some physicians have concerns about antibiotic resistance with this protocol, the rationale for extended antibiotic prophylaxis centers around extending the "golden period" for maintaining low microbe levels and therefore preventing periprosthetic joint infection in TJA [23, 25]. Further, the choice of wound dressing should be considered as the use of closed incision negative pressure wound therapy may be beneficial in reducing the incidence of incisional wound complications in high-risk patients [26].

Barriers to Early Discharge in TJA

After successful patient selection and optimization, identifying the barriers to rapid discharge for outpatient TJA patients are of utmost importance for continual protocol improvements. Recent studies suggest the main predictors for patients not discharging same-day or next-day are postoperative urinary retention (POUR) [27]; hypotension, intractable pain, and nausea [28, 29]; general motor weakness [29]; and hypoxemia [3] among others. Further study is necessary to elucidate these predictors and other barriers to early discharge in TJA.

Conclusion

In summary, outpatient TJA is expected to increase exponentially over the next decade which makes medical evaluation and patient selection paramount for its continued success. Several medical risk stratification tools exist but are limited by low scientific precision and were designed to evaluate medical risk rather than surgical risk to rapid discharge following TJA. The OARA Score was specifically designed to screen for patients who are surgically appropriate for outpatient TJA and accounts for comorbidities in nine medical categories. Furthermore, perioperative patient optimization with multidisciplinary team protocols, proper intraoperative fluid management, and multimodal pain control is also critical to a successful outpatient TJA program.

References

1. Lan RH, Samuel LT, Grits D, Kamath AF. Contemporary outpatient arthroplasty is safe compared with inpatient surgery: a propensity score-matched analysis of 574,375 procedures. J Bone Joint Surg Am. 2021;103:593–600. https://doi.org/10.2106/JBJS.20.01307.
2. Pollock M, Somerville L, Firth A, Lanting B. Outpatient Total hip arthroplasty, total knee arthroplasty, and unicompartmental knee arthroplasty: a systematic review of the literature. JBJS Rev. 2016;4:e4. https://doi.org/10.2106/JBJS.RVW.16.00002.
3. Deans CF, Buller LT, Ziemba-Davis M, Meneghini RM. Same-day discharge following aseptic revision and conversion total joint arthroplasty: a single-institution experience. Arthroplasty Today. 2022;17:159–64. https://doi.org/10.1016/j.artd.2022.07.022.
4. Crawford DA, Lombardi AV, Berend KR, Morris MJ, Adams JB. The feasibility of outpatient conversion and revision hip arthroplasty in selected patients. Hip Int J Clin Exp Res Hip Pathol Ther. 2021;31:393–7. https://doi.org/10.1177/1120700019894949.
5. Law JI, Adams JB, Berend KR, Lombardi AV, Crawford DA. The feasibility of outpatient revision total knee arthroplasty in selected case scenarios. J Arthroplast. 2020;35:S92–6. https://doi.org/10.1016/j.arth.2020.02.021.
6. Gu A, Gerhard EF, Wei C, Bovonratwet P, Stake S, Sculco PK, et al. Aseptic revision total knee can be performed as part of a short-stay arthroplasty program: an analysis of the National Surgical Quality Improvement Program Database. J Knee Surg. 2021;34:764–71. https://doi.org/10.1055/s-0039-3400539.
7. Dyrda L. 16 things to know about outpatient total joint replacements and ASCs 2017.
8. Owens WD, Felts JA, Spitznagel EL. ASA physical status classifications: a study of consistency of ratings. Anesthesiology. 1978;49:239–43. https://doi.org/10.1097/00000542-197810000-00003.
9. Charlson ME, Pompei P, Ales KL, MacKenzie CR. A new method of classifying prognostic comorbidity in longitudinal studies: development and validation. J Chronic Dis. 1987;40:373–83. https://doi.org/10.1016/0021-9681(87)90171-8.
10. Oldmeadow LB, McBurney H, Robertson VJ. Predicting risk of extended inpatient rehabilitation after hip or knee arthroplasty. J Arthroplast. 2003;18:775–9. https://doi.org/10.1016/s0883-5403(03)00151-7.
11. Meneghini RM, Ziemba-Davis M, Ishmael MK, Kuzma AL, Caccavallo P. Safe selection of outpatient joint arthroplasty patients with medical risk stratification: the "Outpatient Arthroplasty Risk Assessment Score". J Arthroplast. 2017;32:2325–31. https://doi.org/10.1016/j.arth.2017.03.004.
12. Ziemba-Davis M, Caccavallo P, Meneghini RM. Outpatient joint arthroplasty-patient selection: update on the outpatient arthroplasty risk assessment score. J Arthroplast. 2019;34:S40–3. https://doi.org/10.1016/j.arth.2019.01.007.
13. Kim KY, Feng JE, Anoushiravani AA, Dranoff E, Davidovitch RI, Schwarzkopf R. Rapid discharge in total hip arthroplasty: utility of the outpatient arthroplasty risk assessment tool in predicting same-day and next-day discharge. J Arthroplast. 2018;33:2412–6. https://doi.org/10.1016/j.arth.2018.03.025.
14. Levine B, Caccavallo P, Springer B, Meneghini RM. Postoperative patient treatment for total knee arthroplasty. Instr Course Lect. 2018;67:241–51.
15. Miller TE, Myles PS. Perioperative fluid therapy for major surgery. Anesthesiology. 2019;130:825–32. https://doi.org/10.1097/ALN.0000000000002603.

16. Goode VM, Morgan B, Muckler VC, Cary MP, Zdeb CE, Zychowicz M. Multimodal pain management for major joint replacement surgery. Orthop Nurs. 2019;38:150–6. https://doi.org/10.1097/NOR.0000000000000525.
17. Ma H-H, Chou T-FA, Tsai S-W, Chen C-F, Wu P-K, Chen W-M. The efficacy of intraoperative periarticular injection in total hip arthroplasty: a systematic review and meta-analysis. BMC Musculoskelet Disord. 2019;20:269. https://doi.org/10.1186/s12891-019-2628-7.
18. Sreedharan Nair V, Ganeshan Radhamony N, Rajendra R, Mishra R. Effectiveness of intraoperative periarticular cocktail injection for pain control and knee motion recovery after total knee replacement. Arthroplast Today. 2019;5:320–4. https://doi.org/10.1016/j.artd.2019.05.004.
19. Benoni G, Fredin H. Fibrinolytic inhibition with tranexamic acid reduces blood loss and blood transfusion after knee arthroplasty: a prospective, randomised, double-blind study of 86 patients. J Bone Joint Surg (Br). 1996;78:434–40.
20. Kayupov E, Fillingham YA, Okroj K, Plummer DR, Moric M, Gerlinger TL, et al. Oral and intravenous tranexamic acid are equivalent at reducing blood loss following total hip arthroplasty: a randomized controlled trial. J Bone Joint Surg Am. 2017;99:373–8. https://doi.org/10.2106/JBJS.16.00188.
21. Licini DJ, Meneghini RM. Modern abbreviated computer navigation of the femur reduces blood loss in total knee arthroplasty. J Arthroplast. 2015;30:1729–32. https://doi.org/10.1016/j.arth.2015.04.020.
22. Inabathula A, Dilley JE, Ziemba-Davis M, Warth LC, Azzam KA, Ireland PH, et al. Extended Oral antibiotic prophylaxis in high-risk patients substantially reduces primary total hip and knee arthroplasty 90-day infection rate. J Bone Joint Surg Am. 2018;100:2103–9. https://doi.org/10.2106/JBJS.17.01485.
23. Kheir MM, Dilley JE, Ziemba-Davis M, Meneghini RM. The AAHKS clinical research award: extended Oral antibiotics prevent periprosthetic joint infection in high-risk cases: 3855 patients with 1-year follow-up. J Arthroplast. 2021;36:S18–25. https://doi.org/10.1016/j.arth.2021.01.051.
24. Zingg M, Kheir MM, Ziemba-Davis M, Meneghini RM. Reduced infection rate after aseptic revision total knee arthroplasty with extended Oral antibiotic protocol. J Arthroplast. 2022;37:905–9. https://doi.org/10.1016/j.arth.2022.01.040.
25. Illingworth KD, Mihalko WM, Parvizi J, Sculco T, McArthur B, el Bitar Y, et al. How to minimize infection and thereby maximize patient outcomes in total joint arthroplasty: a multicenter approach: AAOS exhibit selection. J Bone Joint Surg Am. 2013;95:e50. https://doi.org/10.2106/JBJS.L.00596.
26. Doman DM, Young AM, Buller LT, Deckard ER, Meneghini RM. Comparison of surgical site complications with negative pressure wound therapy vs silver impregnated dressing in high-risk total knee arthroplasty patients: a matched cohort study. J Arthroplast. 2021;36:3437–42. https://doi.org/10.1016/j.arth.2021.05.030.
27. Ziemba-Davis M, Nielson M, Kraus K, Duncan N, Nayyar N, Meneghini RM. Identifiable risk factors to minimize postoperative urinary retention in modern outpatient rapid recovery total joint arthroplasty. J Arthroplast. 2019;34:S343–7. https://doi.org/10.1016/j.arth.2019.03.015.
28. Hoffmann JD, Kusnezov NA, Dunn JC, Zarkadis NJ, Goodman GP, Berger RA. The shift to same-day outpatient joint arthroplasty: a systematic review. J Arthroplast. 2018;33:1265–74. https://doi.org/10.1016/j.arth.2017.11.027.
29. Bodrogi A, Dervin GF, Beaulé PE. Management of patients undergoing same-day discharge primary total hip and knee arthroplasty. CMAJ Can Med Assoc J. 2020;192:E34–9. https://doi.org/10.1503/cmaj.190182.

Chapter 2
Medical Optimization and Risk Mitigation for Readmission

Vignesh K. Alamanda and Bryan D. Springer

Introduction

Primary total joint arthroplasty (TJA) represents one of the most commonly performed surgeries in the United States. Rates of outpatient TJA have dramatically increased [1] and while studies have shown that appropriately selected patients undergoing outpatient TJA have similar outcomes to standard-stay inpatients, it is crucial that these patients are optimized prior to their surgical intervention to ensure safe and timely discharge [2, 3].

Modifiable Versus Non-modifiable Risk Factors

Risk factors can be differentiated between modifiable and non-modifiable. A modifiable risk factor is one that can be changed, and such change can result in a different outcome for that patient. A non-modifiable risk factor is one that cannot be changed and, although important to recognize and counsel the patient on, is unfortunately beyond the control of the surgeon and their patients. This chapter will focus on identifying and acting on modifiable risk factors.

V. K. Alamanda
Hospital for Special Surgery, New York, NY, USA

B. D. Springer (✉)
Hospital for Special Surgery, New York, NY, USA

OrthoCarolina Hip and Knee Center, Charlotte, NC, USA
e-mail: Bryan.springer@orthocarolina.com

R. M. Meneghini, L. T. Buller (eds.), *Outpatient Hip and Knee Replacement*,
https://doi.org/10.1007/978-3-031-27037-6_2

Patient Modifiable Risk Factors and Current Evidence

Diabetes

Diabetes and poor glycemic control have not only been associated with an increased risk of surgical site infection but it is also implicated as a major contributor to PJI in multiple studies. Analysis of these studies has shown a diagnosis of diabetes increases the odds of PJI by more than double [4]. Hemoglobin A1c (Hgb A1c) has been used as a marker of glycemic control in TJA candidates. A simple blood test, Hgb A1c, provides insight into a patient's glycemic control over the past 3 months [5]. Patients with good glycemic control have a Hgb A1C level of less than 7.0%. Other markers of glycemic control include perioperative glucose levels, which some feel better predict PJI when compared to Hgb A1c alone [6]. Additionally, serum fructosamine has been suggested as an adjunct measure of glycemic control over a shorter duration of time when compared to Hgb A1c [7, 8].

Physiologically, the stress from surgery results in an increased production of hormones that antagonize insulin and predispose patients to a relative hyperglycemic state. Thus, in patients with already impaired glycemic control, it is crucial that perioperative control be strictly enforced. Postoperative hyperglycemia, even in patients without a diagnosis of diabetes, can increase the risk of developing a surgical site infection in a dose-related manner. Thus, it is the recommendation of the authors that blood glucose levels be maintained between 110 and180 mg/dL (optimal cutoff of around137 mg/dL) [9] in the perioperative period through frequent blood sugar checks and initiation of diabetic management protocols postoperatively following primary TJA [9]. We also recommend postponing surgery in patients with uncontrolled diabetes and encouraging them to work with their primary care provider, a nutritionist, and/or an endocrinologist on better glycemic control.

Obesity

Obesity is when a person is too heavy for their height. Obesity is a global pandemic thought to be caused by people consuming foods and drinks that are more energy-dense (high in sugars and fats), and engaging in less physical activity. Body mass index (BMI) is an index of weight-for-height used to classify obesity. It is defined as a person's weight in kilograms divided by the square of their height in meters (kg/m^2). In adults, overweight is defined as a BMI of 25 or more, whereas obesity is a BMI of 30 or more.

Obesity has been correlated with higher rates of osteoarthritis and eventually increased utilization of TJA [10]. Studies have shown that patient satisfaction and functional improvement among the obese patient population is similar to the non-obese group following TJA. However, obese patients are at a higher risk of postoperative complications [11]. Obesity predisposes patients to an increased surgical dissection during exposure of the arthritic joint being replaced. This, in turn, can lead to longer surgical times, which is associated with a higher risk of PJI [12]. The poor vascularity of adipose tissue further compounds this problem, leading to poor wound healing and a higher risk of persistent wound drainage. A consensus opinion from the American Association of Hip and Knee Surgeons (AAHKS) evidence-based committee emphasized considering delaying elective TJA in patients with a BMI > 40 kg/m^2, especially when associated with other comorbid conditions [10]. Additionally, some obese patients have metabolic syndrome, which is a cluster of conditions arising from insulin resistance that impairs normal leukocyte function. It is defined as having a BMI > 30 kg/m^2 with central obesity, as well as two of the following: hyperlipidemia, hyperglyceridemia, hypertension, or diabetes [13]. Zmistowski et al. demonstrated an increased risk of PJI (14.3% vs 0.8%) in those with uncontrolled metabolic syndrome when compared to a healthy cohort [14]. Thus, patients with obesity should be screened for other characteristics that may define metabolic syndrome and consideration should be made to counsel these patients on the importance of modification of some or all of these risk factors.

Malnutrition

Malnutrition is often an unrecognized aspect of obesity, associated with the consumption of high caloric but nutritionally poor diets. Malnutrition was found to be present in 42.9% of obese patients in a prospective study evaluating the role of malnutrition in TJA patients [15]. Laboratory tests can help to identify patients at risk for malnutrition. These include a total lymphocyte count of less than 1500 cells/mm^3, a serum albumin of less than 3.5 g/dL, or a transferrin level of less than 200 mg/ dL. Patients with preoperative malnutrition should be encouraged to work with a dietician to help improve their nutritional intake and help prepare them for the catabolic demands required in the postsurgical period.

Smoking

Smoking, and its principal ingredient nicotine, has been associated with decreased oxygen delivery to tissues secondary to microvascular constriction. Duchman et al. reported an increased risk of wound complications with current more so than former smokers in a large national database study [16]. The deleterious effects, in particular PJI, seen with smoking have been confirmed by other studies [17].

Studies have shown smoking cessation programs may decrease complications associated with the use of nicotine, even as late as 4 weeks preoperatively [18]. Thus, we recommend patients considering elective primary TJA have a minimum period of 4 weeks of smoking cessation prior to their surgery. Smoking cessation can be confirmed via easily available laboratory tests such as the serum cotinine assay (normal value of <=10 ng/d).

Vitamin D

Vitamin D plays a crucial role in bone health. Vitamin D deficiency, as defined by a serum 25-hydroxyvitamin D concentration $\leq$ 20 ng/mL, is prevalent in over 40% of the United States population [19]. Interestingly, low levels of Vitamin D have been associated with PJI. Animal models have also shown that the reversal of Vitamin D deficiency can help decrease the development of PJI [20]. Thus, we recommend patients with Vitamin D deficiency begin supplementation preoperatively.

Staphylococcus Aureus Screening

Implementation of an institution wide prescreening program using nasal swab rapid polymerase chain reaction has allowed for the identification of patients who are colonized with *Staphylococcus aureus (S. aureus)* and Methicillin Resistant *S. aureus* (MRSA). Both universal decolonization and selected decolonization of only colonized patients help with the elimination of the bacteria from a patient's nasal flora preoperatively. Nasal decolonization results in a significant reduction in postoperative surgical site infections [21]. We Recommend patients undergoing elective TJA undergo screening for *S. aureus* through nasal swabs and that surgeons consider providing all patients, or just those that are colonized, with mupirocin nasal ointment to be used twice daily in both nares and a bath with chlorhexidine daily for 5 days prior to the scheduled surgery. Additionally, we recommend patients screening positive for MRSA receive a single dose of vancomycin in addition to standard perioperative antibiotics on the day of their surgery.

Inflammatory Arthropathies

Patients afflicted with inflammatory arthropathies such as rheumatoid arthritis and systemic lupus erythematosus are at increased risk of postoperative PJI. Multiple systematic reviews have validated the correlation between inflammatory arthropathies and PJI, with Kong et al. demonstrating rheumatoid arthritis can increase the odds of PJI by 1.6 times [22]. Many patients with inflammatory arthropathies present to their surgeon on immunomodulators. These medications have the potential to significantly impair wound healing and increase the risk of PJI. For example, Momohara et al. demonstrated that patients on Tumor Necrosis Factor (TNF)-alpha inhibitors are at significantly higher risk for surgical site infections [23]. Guidelines jointly published by the American College of Rheumatology (ACR) and the American Association of Hip and Knee Surgeon (AAHKS) used available evidence to make recommendations on which medications should be continued and which medications should be stopped in elective TJA [24]. In general, traditional Disease Modifying Antirheumatic Medications (DMARDS) do not need to be withheld prior to surgery. However, immunomodulating agents, such as TNF-alpha inhibitors, place patients at increased risk for the development of a PJI and should be withheld one dosing cycle prior to surgery.

Antibiotic Prophylaxis

Preoperative antibiotic prophylaxis is effective in reducing rates of surgical site infections and has been incorporated in many surgical checklists [25]. Routine prophylactic antibiotics should be dosed in accordance with the patient's weight and should include a first-generation cephalosporin such as cefazolin. Patients allergic to beta-lactam antibiotics should receive vancomycin or clindamycin in a timely fashion. Prophylactic antibiotics should be administered ideally as close to the time of the incision as possible. First-generation cephalosporin and clindamycin should be administered within 1 h and vancomycin should be administered within 2 h of incision. We recommend that a single dose of vancomycin be considered in addition to standard preoperative antibiotics for those who have been shown to be colonized with MRSA or those who had a prior infection with MRSA.

Conclusion

The well-known saying, a stitch in time saves nine, is certainly applicable to improving outcomes and decreasing rates of complications among patients undergoing outpatient TJA. While it will never be possible to completely eliminate all risks, it can certainly help improve the odds.

References

1. Krause A, Sayeed Z, El-Othmani M, Pallekonda V, Mihalko W, Saleh KJ. Outpatient Total knee arthroplasty: are we there yet? (part 1). Orthop Clin North Am. 2018;49(1):1–6.
2. Bert JM, Hooper J, Moen S. Outpatient Total joint arthroplasty. Curr Rev Musculoskelet Med. 2017;10(4):567–74.
3. Lovett-Carter D, Sayeed Z, Abaab L, Pallekonda V, Mihalko W, Saleh KJ. Impact of outpatient Total joint replacement on postoperative outcomes. Orthop Clin North Am. 2018;49(1):35–44.

4. Marchant MH Jr, Viens NA, Cook C, Vail TP, Bolognesi MP. The impact of glycemic control and diabetes mellitus on perioperative outcomes after total joint arthroplasty. J Bone Joint Surg Am. 2009;91(7):1621–9.
5. Stryker LS, Abdel MP, Morrey ME, Morrow MM, Kor DJ, Morrey BF. Elevated postoperative blood glucose and preoperative hemoglobin A1C are associated with increased wound complications following total joint arthroplasty. J Bone Joint Surg Am. 2013;95(9):808–14. S1–2
6. Iorio R, Williams KM, Marcantonio AJ, Specht LM, Tilzey JF, Healy WL. Diabetes mellitus, hemoglobin A1C, and the incidence of total joint arthroplasty infection. J Arthroplast. 2012;27(5):726–9 e1.
7. Shohat N, Tarabichi M, Tischler EH, Jabbour S, Parvizi J. Serum Fructosamine: a simple and inexpensive test for assessing preoperative glycemic control. J Bone Joint Surg Am. 2017;99(22):1900–8.
8. Kheir MM, Tan TL, Kheir M, Maltenfort MG, Chen AF. Postoperative blood glucose levels predict infection after Total joint arthroplasty. J Bone Joint Surg Am. 2018;100(16):1423–31.
9. Gallagher JM, Erich RA, Gattermeyer R, Beam KK. Postoperative hyperglycemia can be safely and effectively controlled in both diabetic and nondiabetic patients with use of a subcutaneous insulin protocol. JB JS Open Access. 2017;2(1):e0008.
10. Workgroup of the American Association of H, Knee Surgeons Evidence Based C. Obesity and total joint arthroplasty: a literature based review. J Arthroplast. 2013;28(5):714–21.
11. Mason JB, Callaghan JJ, Hozack WJ, Krebs V, Mont MA, Parvizi J. Obesity in total joint arthroplasty: an issue with gravity. J Arthroplast. 2014;29(10):1879.
12. Wang Q, Goswami K, Shohat N, Aalirezaie A, Manrique J, Parvizi J. Longer operative time results in a higher rate of subsequent Periprosthetic joint infection in patients undergoing primary joint arthroplasty. J Arthroplast. 2019;34(5):947–53. https://doi.org/10.1016/j.arth.2019.01.027. Epub 2019 Jan 18
13. Gage MJ, Schwarzkopf R, Abrouk M, Slover JD. Impact of metabolic syndrome on perioperative complication rates after total joint arthroplasty surgery. J Arthroplast. 2014;29(9):1842–5.
14. Zmistowski B, Dizdarevic I, Jacovides CL, Radcliff KE, Mraovic B, Parvizi J. Patients with uncontrolled components of metabolic syndrome have increased risk of complications following total joint arthroplasty. J Arthroplast. 2013;28(6):904–7.
15. Huang R, Greenky M, Kerr GJ, Austin MS, Parvizi J. The effect of malnutrition on patients undergoing elective joint arthroplasty. J Arthroplast. 2013;28(8 Suppl):21–4.
16. Duchman KR, Gao Y, Pugely AJ, Martin CT, Noiseux NO, Callaghan JJ. The effect of smoking on short-term complications following Total hip and knee arthroplasty. J Bone Joint Surg Am. 2015;97(13):1049–58.
17. Teng S, Yi C, Krettek C, Jagodzinski M. Smoking and risk of prosthesis-related complications after total hip arthroplasty: a meta-analysis of cohort studies. PLoS One. 2015;10(4):e0125294.
18. Lindstrom D, Sadr Azodi O, Wladis A, Tonnesen H, Linder S, Nasell H, et al. Effects of a perioperative smoking cessation intervention on postoperative complications: a randomized trial. Ann Surg. 2008;248(5):739–45.
19. Forrest KY, Stuhldreher WL. Prevalence and correlates of vitamin D deficiency in US adults. Nutr Res. 2011;31(1):48–54.
20. Hegde V, Dworsky EM, Stavrakis AI, Loftin AH, Zoller SD, Park HY, et al. Single-dose, preoperative vitamin-D supplementation decreases infection in a mouse model of periprosthetic joint infection. J Bone Joint Surg Am. 2017;99(20):1737–44.
21. Kim DH, Spencer M, Davidson SM, Li L, Shaw JD, Gulczynski D, et al. Institutional prescreening for detection and eradication of methicillin-resistant Staphylococcus aureus in patients undergoing elective orthopaedic surgery. J Bone Joint Surg Am. 2010;92(9):1820–6.
22. Kong L, Cao J, Zhang Y, Ding W, Shen Y. Risk factors for periprosthetic joint infection following primary total hip or knee arthroplasty: a meta-analysis. Int Wound J. 2017;14(3):529–36.
23. Momohara S, Kawakami K, Iwamoto T, Yano K, Sakuma Y, Hiroshima R, et al. Prosthetic joint infection after total hip or knee arthroplasty in rheumatoid arthritis patients treated

with nonbiologic and biologic disease-modifying antirheumatic drugs. Mod Rheumatol. 2011;21(5):469–75.
24. Goodman SM, Springer B, Guyatt G, Abdel MP, Dasa V, George M, et al. 2017 American College of Rheumatology/American Association of hip and Knee Surgeons Guideline for the perioperative Management of Antirheumatic Medication in patients with rheumatic diseases undergoing elective Total hip or Total knee arthroplasty. J Arthroplast. 2017;32(9):2628–38.
25. Fernandez AH, Monge V, Garcinuno MA. Surgical antibiotic prophylaxis: effect in postoperative infections. Eur J Epidemiol. 2001;17(4):369–74.

Chapter 3
Surgical Appropriateness for Outpatient TJA in an ASC

Jesua Law, David A. Crawford, and Adolf V. Lombardi

Introduction

Outpatient Total Joint Arthroplasty (TJA) is the future [1]. Over the last decade there have been multiple advancements in multimodal pain control [2, 3], blood management [4], minimally invasive surgical techniques, and rapid recovery protocols [5–7] that have revolutionized joint replacement surgery. These advancements have changed the length of stay from weeks to days, and recently to only a few hours at an outpatient setting [8, 9]. Higher patient satisfaction scores [10] and fewer complications [11] have been documented in the outpatient setting as patients are able to recover in an environment familiar to them, safe from pathogens [12], and unnecessary lab draws [13]. With benefits to the patient, surgeon, and health-care system, outpatient TJA has gained popularity worldwide [14]. The Centers for Medicare and Medicaid Services (CMS) has seen the benefits of this and removed primary total hip and knee arthroplasty from the inpatient-only list, as well as allowing these procedures to be performed at an ASC.

Ambulatory Surgery Center Versus the Hospital

After acknowledging the benefits of outpatient TJA, the next decision is the surgical venue for the operation. Surgeons have the option of performing surgery at a free-standing hospital under an admitted "inpatient" status, a hospital-based "outpatient" setting, or an ASC. While not all patients are candidates for a procedure at an ASC,

J. Law (✉) · D. A. Crawford · A. V. Lombardi
JIS Orthopedics, New Albany, OH, USA
e-mail: lawji@joint-surgeons.com; crawfordda@joint-surgeons.com; lombardiav@joint-surgeons.com

R. M. Meneghini, L. T. Buller (eds.), *Outpatient Hip and Knee Replacement*,
https://doi.org/10.1007/978-3-031-27037-6_3

the ASC offers several advantages over the other two options. Ambulatory surgery centers usually offer improved proficiency, as the mindset of most team members of the ASC is to maximize productivity and efficiency [15]. Most staff members are cross-trained and able to both provide patient care and assist in turnovers. The enthusiasm to work efficiently is enhanced at an ASC as staff members realize they are able to go home once the work is done and not "waiting for a shift to end." Ambulatory surgery centers usually offer a smaller, more personalized experience for the surgeon and patient, and in physician-owned ASCs the healthcare provider is able to directly impact the patient experience without layers or hospital bureaucracy impeding patient care.

It is important to emphasize that not all patients are candidates for outpatient surgery and not all surgeries should be attempted at an ASC. Patient selection, and case selection, is critically important for ASC cases to achieve the best possible outcomes while minimizing complications.

Selection of Patients

Most patients will be appropriate candidates for outpatient TJA at an ASC; however, some may have medical comorbidities that preclude this environment. Many authors have discussed techniques for determining which patients are appropriate for outpatient surgery [11]. One model uses an outpatient arthroplasty risk assessment (OARA) scoring system [16] to help the surgeon evaluate comorbid conditions and make the decision for outpatient surgery. The OARA scoring system is proprietary and requires a licensing fee. A more simplified model [17] investigates whether the patient has medical comorbid conditions that are not optimized prior to the time of surgery. If chronic comorbid medical conditions are not optimized, then elective surgery should be delayed until these conditions are optimized. In this simplified model, the only contraindication for outpatient surgery is a failing organ system. Patients with Chronic Obstructive Pulmonary Disease (specifically those requiring oxygen), asthma, congestive heart failure, chronic kidney disease, or liver cirrhosis [18] are at the highest risk for needing inpatient hospitalization and outpatient TJA should be cautioned. Surgery in this group of patients should be performed alongside a multidisciplinary medical team in a hospital setting for proper monitoring of the patient. It should be emphasized that inpatient hospitalization is for monitoring the medical comorbid conditions and not due to the arthroplasty itself. Once the proper outpatient is selected, the surgeon must evaluate the limitations of the ASC and consider the following set of conditions outlined below to determine if an ASC is a proper venue.

Selection of Cases

When considering the appropriateness of surgery at an ASC, it is critical that the surgeon considers the complexity of the case, including the limited storage and sterilization capacity. Since streamlined efficiency and steady workflow are the main focus, most primary joint replacement cases can effortlessly be accomplished at an ASC. However, complex revisions can easily overwhelm the sterile processing capabilities when multiple instrument trays are needed. Oftentimes, these cases may not even be candidates for outpatient joint replacement surgery, let alone surgery in the ASC. Inpatient hospitalization should be considered in certain complex cases, such as difficult femoral or acetabular reconstructions or grossly infected cases, due to the greater propensity for blood loss [19] and the need for medical subspecialty consultation. Polyethylene liner exchanges, partial knee to total knee replacement revisions, and single component revisions are just a few of the "simpler" revisions that can be safely performed in an outpatient ASC setting. However, a hospital-based outpatient surgery center, or even inpatient hospitalization, should be considered as the complexity of the case increases.

Educating the Patient

Many patients will have preconceived notions of what to expect from their TJA. Inpatient hospitalization and discharge to a short-term rehabilitation facility is the perceived standard of care for some patients who may have had an arthroplasty years ago or know a family member who underwent a joint replacement surgery. Among these patients, outpatient surgery at an ASC is a foreign idea and same-day discharge may seem rushed or intimidating. The surgeon and staff should educate the patient regarding the benefits of recovering from surgery at home [20], and the advancements in pain management protocols that allow their recovery to be accomplished comfortably. This explanation eases fears and improves satisfaction and patient compliance [19–21]. A unified message must be delivered to the patient and family so that the patient feels comfortable and supported by all members of the team from the office staff to hospital/ASC employees.

Joint replacement classes, and even simple handouts, are some of the various forms of education available to the patient. Regardless of the messaging, the primary source of educational materials should be written since patients often forget up to 80% of the information presented during the visit [21] and further questions often arise after the clinical encounter. Included in the patient educational materials are expectations regarding wound care and hygiene after the surgical procedure, exercises, and activity of daily living (ADL) goals for the first few days after surgery, as well as a preoperative medical evaluation overview. Physical therapists are available pre- and postoperatively to outline the stepwise approach to safely performing ADLs, to teach patients how to use ambulatory aids, and perform more complex activities such as going up and down stairs. Expectations for pain management, blood clot prevention, presurgical home planning, and an outline of the risks of surgery should all be included in these educational materials.

When questions arise that are not covered in the educational material, knowledgeable office staff should be available to aid in answering questions. By viewing the facility before surgery, patients are able to meet the staff and postoperative care team. Wound and dressing instructions should be explained by knowledgeable nursing staff as well as what signs to look for if problems arise. To improve patient comfort and decrease fear, setting clear expectations between the surgeon, patient, and family [5–7] has been shown to be of prime importance.

Finally, patients should be educated on the fact that an ASC, despite having improved outcomes and decreased complications, has limitations and if complications or difficult situations arise the patient may need to transfer to a free-standing hospital.

Anesthesia and Pain Management

Many patients are fearful of outpatient TJA due to a perceived inability to manage their pain once at home [22]. However, in outpatient TJA, uncontrolled pain is rarely the cause of an overnight stay or emergency room visit within 48 h of surgery [11, 17]. One of the biggest advancements in the ability to perform joint replacement surgery at an ASC is the advent of multimodal pain control and rapid recovery protocols [3, 23–25]. The minimization of pain, sedation, and nausea, while promoting mobilization and a safe discharge, is the prime objective of these rapid recovery protocols and will be discussed in subsequent chapters. Many multimodal pain regimens have been described, but most involve a nonsteroidal anti-inflammatory (NSAID), regional anesthesia, and a non-narcotic analgesic (acetaminophen) preoperatively along with minimal opioid usage.

The transition from general anesthesia alone to regional anesthesia has greatly increased patient comfort and minimized the need for postoperative opioids. In both partial and total knee arthroplasty patients, an adductor canal block and infiltration of anesthetic into the posterior capsule are recommended. Femoral nerve blocks should be avoided in the ASC setting due to quadriceps muscle weakness and increased fall risk [26–28]. In hip replacement patients, spinal anesthesia in combination with sedation or light general anesthesia has been shown to decrease blood loss, decrease short-term complications, lead to fewer "nonhome" discharges, and improve patient satisfaction [29] when compared to general anesthesia alone [30]. Narcotics should be avoided in regional anesthesia blocks due to pruritus, nausea, and sedation, which all can result in the patient staying more than 23 h for observation. Prior to closure, it is recommended that the patient receive an infiltration of local anesthesia into the periarticular tissue, which has been shown to decrease postoperative pain [31]. This combination of peripheral and general anesthesia has been shown to decrease pain, increase early mobility, decrease the need for narcotics, decrease the length of stay, and reduce readmissions [32, 33].

Postoperative Care and Follow Up

Postoperatively, the patient should have clear goals and expectations as outlined above in the patient education section. It is important that the patient feels empowered to perform their ADLs, but not abandoned. Oftentimes, a call from a staff member shortly after surgery helps remind the patient of the predetermined goals that were expressed and keeps the patient on track, answers questions, and helps determine what is "normal and abnormal" with recovery. Physical therapy should be started shortly after surgery to coach the patient in performing ADLs safely. The goal of the therapist is to ensure a smooth transition to independence as well as keep a trained eye on the patient to ensure issues do not arise. Therapists who see many postsurgical patients can be a great resource for the patient, and the surgeon, by alerting a member of the surgical team if concerns arise before issues escalate and also keep the patient from feeling abandoned in the postoperative recovery period.

Follow-up visits vary from institution and clinical practice, but often require the patient to come in for a wound check, postoperative radiograph, and range of motion evaluation. If issues arise in this time period there may be a role to increase physical therapy for a period of time and/or schedule a manipulation under anesthesia.

23-Hour Observation and Transfer Agreements

Surgery at an ASC has many benefits, as listed above, but also some limitations. In a recent 2018 publication [17], 94% of total hip replacement patients were able to discharge home as planned. Of the patients that required an overnight stay, half were due to convenience and the most common medical reason for overnight observation was urinary retention. Total knee patients had a higher overnight observation for medical necessity at 7.6% [11]. Not every state allows for 23-h observation at the ASC and the facility should have plans in place in case the patient necessitates a longer than expected stay.

Patients who need further evaluation, blood transfusions, or have unforeseen medical complications, while rare [11, 17], may require a short observational period at an inpatient hospital setting. This is never convenient for the patient or family, but having plans in place eases anxiety. In these situations, the ASC should have a transfer agreement with a nearby hospital allowing patients direct access to a higher level of medical care. It is important the patient receive discharge materials, prescriptions, and any medical equipment needed postoperatively and the surgeon be in communication with the admitting medical provider.

Conclusion

Outpatient joint replacement surgery at an ASC is safe, efficient, and has low complication rates. In the properly selected patient, joint replacement surgery at an ASC can have benefits to the surgeon and patient while being more cost-effective to the healthcare system as a whole.

References

1. Berend ME, Lackey W, Carter J. Outpatient-focused joint arthroplasty is the future: the midwest center for joint replacement experience. J Arthroplasty. 2018;33(6):1647–8.
2. Berend ME, Berend KR, Lombardi AV Jr. Advances in pain management: game changers in knee arthroplasty. Bone Joint J. 2014;96-B(11 Supple A):7–9.
3. Berger RA, Sanders SA, Thill ES, et al. Newer anesthesia and rehabilitation protocols enable outpatient hip replacement in selected patients. Clin Orthop Relat Res. 2009;467(6):1424–30.
4. Krauss ES, Cronin M, Suratwala SJ, et al. Use of intravenous tranexamic acid improves early ambulation after total knee arthroplasty and anterior and posterior total hip arthroplasty. Am J Orthop (Belle Mead NJ). 2017;46(5):E314–9.
5. Berend KR, Lombardi AV Jr. Mallory TH: rapid recovery protocol for peri-operative care of total hip and total knee arthroplasty patients. Surg Technol Int. 2004;13:239–47.
6. Lombardi AV Jr, Viacava AJ, Berend KR. Rapid recovery protocols and minimally invasive surgery help achieve high knee flexion. Clin Orthop Relat Res. 2006;452:117–22.
7. Lombardi AV, Berend KR. Adams JB: a rapid recovery program: early home and pain free. Orthopedics. 2010;33(9):656.
8. Teeny SM, York SC, Benson C, Perdue ST. Does shortened length of hospital stay affect total knee arthroplasty rehabilitation outcomes? J Arthroplast. 2005;20(7 suppl 3):39–45.
9. Cleary PD, Greenfield S, Mulley AG, et al. Variations in length of stay and outcomes for six medical and surgical conditions in Massachusetts and California. JAMA. 1991;266(1):73–9.
10. Kelly MP, Calkins TE, Culvern C, et al. Inpatient versus outpatient hip and knee arthroplasty: which has higher patient satisfaction? J Arthroplast. 2018;33(11):3402–6.
11. Crawford DA, Adams JB, Berend KR, et al. Low complication rates in outpatient total knee arthroplasty. Knee Surg Sports Traumatol Arthrosc. 2019;28(5):1458–64. https://doi.org/10.1007/s00167-019-05538-8.
12. Giuliano KK, Baker D, Quinn B. The epidemiology of nonventilator hospital-acquired pneumonia in the United States. Am J Infect Control. 2018 Mar;46(3):322–7.
13. Greco NJ, Manocchio AG, Lombardi AV, et al. Should postoperative hemoglobin and potassium levels be checked routinely following blood-conserving primary total joint arthroplasty? Bone Joint J. 2019;101-B(1_Supple_A):25–31.
14. Tingle C, Berger RA, Bolognesi MP, et al. Same-day outpatient TJR gains popularity, but careful considerations must be made. Orthopedics Today. 2015;35(8):10–1.
15. Imran JB, Madni TD, Taveras LR, et al. Analysis of operating room efficiency between a hospital-owned ambulatory surgical center and hospital outpatient department. Am J Surg. 2019;218(5):809–12. https://doi.org/10.1016/j.amjsurg.2019.04.017.
16. Meneghini RM, Ziemba-Davis M, Ishmael MK, et al. Safe selection of outpatient joint arthroplasty patients with medical risk stratification: the "outpatient arthroplasty risk assessment score". J Arthroplast. 2017 Aug;32(8):2325–31.
17. Berend KR, Lombardi AV, Berend ME, Adams JB, Morris MJ. Outpatient total hip arthroplasty: a paradigm change. JBJS. 2018;100-B(1 Supple A):31–5.

18. Meding JB, Klay M, Healy A, Ritter MA, Keating EM, Berend ME. The prescreening history and physical in elective total joint arthroplasty. J Arthroplast. 2007;22(6, suppl 2):21–3.
19. Bozic KJ, Katz P, Cisternas M, et al. Hospital resource utilization for primary and revision total hip arthroplasty. J Bone Joint Surg Am. 2005 Mar;87(3):570–6.
20. Dowsey MM, Kilgour ML, Santamaria NM, et al. Clinical pathways in hip and knee arthroplasty: a prospective randomized controlled study. Med J Aust. 1999;170(2):59–62.
21. Kessels R. Patients memory for medical information. J R Soc Med. 2003;96(10):520.
22. Adelani MA, Barrack RL. Patient perceptions of the safety of outpatient total knee arthroplasty. J Arthroplast. 2019;34(3):462–4.
23. Berend KR, Lombardi AV Jr. Liberal indications for minimally invasive oxford unicondylar arthroplasty provide rapid functional recovery and pain relief. Surg Technol Int. 2007;16:193–7.
24. Mears DC, Mears SC, Chelly JE, Dai F, Vulakovich KL. THA with a minimally invasive technique, multi-modal anesthesia, and home rehabilitation: factors associated with early discharge? Clin Orthop Relat Res. 2009;467(6):1412–7.
25. Sculco PK, Pagnano MW. Perioperative solutions for rapid recovery joint arthroplasty: get ahead and stay ahead. J Arthroplast. 2015;30(4):518–20.
26. Sharma S, Iorio R, Specht LM, Davies-Lepie S, Healy WL, et al. Clin Orthop Relat Res. 2010;468(1):135–40.
27. Jaeger P, Nielsen ZJ, Henningsen MH, Hilsted KL, Mathiesen O, Dahl JB. Adductor canal block versus femoral nerve block and quadriceps strength: a randomized, double-blind, placebo-controlled, crossover study in healthy volunteers. Anesthesiology. 2013;118(2):409–15.
28. Sankineani SR, Reddy ARC, Eachempati K, Jangle A, Reddy AV. Comparision of adductor canal block and IPACK block with adductor canal alone after total knee arthroplasty: a prospective control trial on pain and knee function in immediate postoperative period. Eur J Orthop Surg Traumatol. 2018;28:1391–5.
29. Johnson RL, Kopp SL, Burkle CM, et al. Neuraxial vs general anaesthesia for total hip and total knee arthroplasty: a systematic review of comparative- effectiveness research. Br J Anaesth. 2016;116:163–76.
30. MacFarlane AJR, Arun Prasad G, Chan VWS, Brull R. Does regional anesthesia improve outcome after total knee arthroplasty? Clin Orthop Relat Res. 2009;467:2379–402.
31. Lombardi AV Jr, Berend KR, Mallory TH, Dodds KL, Adams JB. Soft tissue and intra-articular injection of bupivacaine, epinephrine, and morphine has a beneficial effect after total knee arthroplasty. Clin Orthop Relat Res. 2004;428:125–30.
32. Beaupre LA, Johnston DB, Dieleman S, Tsui B. Impact of a preemptive multimodal analgesia plus femoral nerve blockade protocol on rehabilitation, hospital length of stay, and postoperative analgesia after primary total knee arthroplasty: a controlled clinical pilot study. Sci World J. 2012;2012:273821.
33. Lovald ST, Ong KL, Lau EC, Joshi GP, Kurtz SM, Malkani AL. Readmission and complications for catheter and injection femoral nerve block administration after total knee arthroplasty in the Medicare population. J Arthroplast. 2015;30(12):2076–81.

Chapter 4
Essential Components of Preoperative Education and Planning

Alexander Sah

Introduction

In recent years, the practice of total joint arthroplasty (TJA) has experienced a dramatic change in environment, both figuratively and literally. In the reimbursement arena, performing TJA in the traditional fee-for-service model has shifted to alternative payment models where surgeons are the leaders in directing the episode of care. As a consequence of this change, surgeons must expand their skills beyond the operating room and coordinate the entire continuum of care to optimize healthcare value. Furthermore, the location of TJA is literally moving away from the traditional hospital setting to freestanding ambulatory surgery centers (ASCs). These figurative and literal changes require adaptations of standard perioperative programs to advanced protocols in order to maximize outcomes and cost savings. Preoperative education has been a mainstay of traditional TJA programs and is even more important for success in these changing environments.

Influence of Bundled Payments on the Patient Experience

Bundled payment models aim to align surgeons and hospitals by placing them at risk for financial penalty if predetermined outcome measures are not achieved. Consequently, new opportunities have arisen where gainsharing relationships are allowed for participants to share in program cost savings. Incentives now motivate surgeon and hospitals to optimize outcomes while minimizing costs [1]. Shifting care and costs away from unnecessary postsurgery treatment services to preoperative education and preparation can achieve many of these goals.

A. Sah (✉)
Institute for Joint Restoration, Washington Hospital, Fremont, CA, USA

R. M. Meneghini, L. T. Buller (eds.), *Outpatient Hip and Knee Replacement*, https://doi.org/10.1007/978-3-031-27037-6_4

The content of preoperative education typically includes general information related to presurgical processes, the surgical procedure, discharge disposition, postoperative care, potential surgical and nonsurgical complications, answers to frequently asked questions, postoperative pain management, and important staff contacts. The adoption of alternative payment models, which include outcomes up to several months after surgery, has led to changes in patient education needs. The success of bundled payment models depends on avoiding adverse events, while minimizing costs, and simultaneously optimizing patient outcomes. Preoperative education can preemptively address many of the common causes for patient adverse events and readmissions thereby making preoperative preparation efforts essential to optimize the overall bundle.

Analyzing the components of the episode of care reveals that the major cost drivers for hip and knee replacement are hospital length of stay (LOS), discharge to post-acute care facilities, and hospital readmission [2, 3]. Literature has shown that discharges to skilled nursing facilities lead to poorer overall outcomes, increased costs, and higher complication rates [4–7]. In the bundled payment environment, standard inpatient joint replacement discharges must be aimed at going home safely to minimize costs and potential complications [8]. Preoperative education classes have shown potential cost savings averaging over $4000 (27.2%) less than total costs for those patients who did not participate in preoperative education classes prior to elective hip or knee replacement [9, 10]. Recent literature has described some of the steps necessary to successfully accomplish these objectives [11–13]. Most of these reports have concluded that preoperative education plays a critical role to achieve these goals [14–18]. Cost savings resulting from proper education can be significant, up to $12,000 per year for those patients who attended an education program prior to surgery [19]. Simply put, preparation efforts prior to surgery pays dividends for cost containment and better outcomes after elective hip and knee replacement surgery.

Traditional Preoperative Joint Replacement Education

While hip and knee replacement are two of the most successful procedures in orthopedics in terms of outcomes and satisfaction, results are improved with optimized perioperative protocols [20]. Most attention is given to those protocols directly affecting the surgical procedure or the immediate pre- or postoperative care provided to the patient. Elements of a successful comprehensive joint replacement program are expansive enough to include all elements of the patient experience, including preoperative education, joint class or camps, office support, and follow-up staff and systems. Although these comprehensive clinical pathway programs are multifaceted, the educational component is one of the most critical pieces for overall success.

Standard educational programs address patient preparation before surgery, the surgical procedure, immediate recovery, avoidance of common complications, and recovery after surgery. To most effectively communicate these issues to patients, traditional preoperative education guidelines suggest simplifying medical terms, using visual aids and models, organizing topics in chronological order, and having presenters be staff who will later interact with the patient again [21]. Education classes located on, or near, the joint replacement floor and at the hospital where surgery will occur allows the opportunity for patient familiarity with the surgical environment. Furthermore, patients and caregivers can become familiar with their route to the hospital, meet staff, and visit the after-surgery areas to reduce anxiety associated with their upcoming surgery.

Prior to surgery, patients learn to optimize their medical health in anticipation of their surgery date. In addition to addressing their individual medical comorbidities before surgery, maximizing overall conditioning and strength can aid in recovery [22]. Furthermore, preparing the home environment for safety and simplifying recovery is beneficial. This focus can greatly improve the chance that patients will feel comfortable being discharged directly home, rather than to a nursing facility. The preoperative class should also explain the surgical procedure in simple terms. The use of videos, visual aids, and actual implant components can help patients understand what is involved in their surgery, and the reasons for the expected recovery. Pain management, swelling control, and ambulation goals are better understood in the context of knowing the surgical procedure. By providing a road map of how to address common symptoms after surgery, the patient is prepared and more confident in the respective treatments. This aspect of preoperative education is critical to avoid emergency room visits and readmissions. Lastly, explanations of the longer term recovery help manage expectations and patient satisfaction.

Thorough educational programs have been shown to benefit patients who attend classes prior to surgery by having less anxiety, better postoperative pain control, more realistic expectations of surgery, and a better understanding of their surgery. Focusing the educational efforts earlier in the surgical experiences has been associated with improved outcomes [23–26]. The benefits of these programs include decreased pre- and postoperative anxiety, decreased postoperative pain, better coping, decreased LOS, increased discharge to home, lower readmissions, and cost savings [27]. Prior studies have shown that comprehensive patient education programs decrease discharge to post-acute care facilities and postoperative complications [28, 29]. Recent data showed that preoperative education as a single intervention decreased LOS following total knee arthroplasty with no increase in complications or readmissions within 90 days of discharge [9]. Furthermore, implementation of patient education has positive impacts upon patient satisfaction, especially in managing pain, which is a leading impediment to early discharge home [30].

The Effect of the Migration Towards Outpatient TJA

Successful outpatient joint replacement relies on building upon an already sound foundation of preoperative education and patient preparation. It is important to understand how the outpatient experience differs from the inpatient experience to best modify existing preoperative education protocols. Outpatient joint replacement differs from standard protocols in only one fundamental way—*time* [31]. It is not defined by different surgical techniques or the use of specific implant types. Outpatient joint replacement simply means having the ability to discharge a patient within a specific time constraint. Once this is understood, the effects of time reduction on the patient experience can be better evaluated.

The most immediate impact of faster discharge is that there is less time to diagnose and treat potential adverse events related to medications, anesthesia, or surgical procedure. Patients and caregivers have less time to address postoperative anxiety or review discharge instructions. Furthermore, recovery from surgery in the outpatient setting is more likely to occur in isolation as opposed to in the inpatient setting. More information must be covered in a shorter period of time for outpatient surgery discharges. Lastly, and possibly most importantly, earlier discharge exposes patients to earlier and more variable postoperative experiences at home. Emphasis needs to be placed on how to manage earlier variability in pain, nausea, swelling, and other symptoms because patients will be at home when some of these may occur for the first time. Expectations for this 6–24 h window after discharge must be clearly explained to the patient and caregiver. For these reasons, a key challenge to the transition from the inpatient to outpatient setting is that the work that traditionally happens after surgery must now occur on the "front-end."

To meet the demands of providing consistent and safe outpatient joint replacement discharges, preoperative education programs must be optimized, and in many cases enhanced beyond standard procedures [32]. By understanding these differences and by being proactive, rather than reactive, the enhanced protocols can provide a safe and successful outpatient experience. In order to prepare for these challenges in outpatient surgery, there are a minimum of four elements of the standard inpatient joint replacement protocols that should be augmented. These areas include preoperative education, discharge instructions, staff availability, and creation of a safety net.

Setting the Foundation of Patient Expectations

The framework for patient expectations and education begins on the initial consultation. The goal of patient and caregiver education is to make patients feel confident managing their own healthcare. Patients should understand that they must take an active role in their success. Preoperative education is important to improve patient expectations prior to surgery and provide them the understanding that they are the primary factor in achieving a good outcome [33]. Preoperative education also prepares patients psychologically for rehabilitation goals by providing them with clear expectations of the recovery process [34]. Providing the patient with adequate information can increase their sense of responsibility for a successful surgery, as well as improve their ability to cope after surgery [35]. It is important that this philosophy of self-empowerment permeates throughout all elements of patient preparation. This understanding is particularly significant because individuals undergoing joint replacement surgery have high expectations for their outcomes [36]. A strong correlation has been reported between patient satisfaction and fulfillment of pain relief and functional restoration [37, 38], Stated another way, up to 20% of all total knee arthroplasty patients are not satisfied with their outcome, and the strongest predictor of dissatisfaction is not having their expectations met [39]. Furthermore, there is a disconnect between patients and surgeons, as patient expectations for pain relief and functional outcome are higher than their surgeons' expectations [40]. Improving the alignment of patient and surgeon expectations before surgery may lead to improved patient satisfaction after joint replacement. The initial consultation and subsequent education programs are critical opportunities to establish this mutual understanding.

Addressing Patient Anxiety Preemptively

As with any elective procedure, patients should be made aware of the potential risks and benefits of surgery. Somewhat unique to TJA are the associated anxieties that patients experience prior to surgery. Patient and caregiver concerns and questions should be thoroughly addressed during the patient education phase. The anxiety of the caregiver must be recognized, as it may also negatively affect the patient [41]. Preoperative education protocols should include written medication instructions, including medications for pain management and venous thromboembolism prophylaxis. A recovery plan should be made, explicitly outlining patient expectations, caregiver responsibilities, and physical therapy or nursing care if needed. Also, patient expectations about pain levels, walking, driving, and returning to work need to be managed and reasonable goals should be established. Some successful programs have included a 2-h presurgery meeting with the patient, a clinical care coordinator, and a physical therapist to outline these expectations and address patient concerns.

Pain after TJA correlates with heightened preoperative anxiety levels [42]. Preoperative education can decrease patient anxiety associated with an upcoming surgical procedure [43, 44]. The literature supports that reducing preoperative patient anxiety results in improved postoperative recovery, leading to higher levels of patient satisfaction with their surgical experience, and reducing levels of self-reported pain up to 1 year after surgery [45]. An observational study reported that 78% of participants believed that preoperative education was responsible for a reduction in their anxiety prior to elective orthopedic surgery [46]. Several studies have evaluated the most effective means to improve patient anxiety prior to surgery and determined that providing information regarding the upcoming surgery and subsequent hospitalization is most beneficial [29, 47, 48].

Understanding Patient Comprehension and Limitations

As education programs become more thorough and more complex, there is a risk that patients will not absorb or retain the information. At some point, increasing the amount of information taught to potentially anxious patients will instead cause more confusion or stress than the benefits it may provide. In these education classes, educators must be aware of the risk of the sheer volume of information conveyed in shortening amounts of time thereby risking overloading the patient. Learners have limitations in how much material they can comprehend, after which, they no longer absorb the information. Worse, there is a risk of causing greater confusion, potentially undermining previous preparation successes. It is also important to be aware of the range of health literacy in the class of attendees. Preoperative education must be taught at the lowest level of patient comprehension so that all participants can benefit [49]. Health literacy remains vital in achieving a patients' understanding of their upcoming surgery and is considered the single best predictor of an individual's health status [50]. Providing education materials at the literacy level of the patient population will improve their understanding of surgery, minimize anxiety, and improve outcomes that are clinically significant [51]. Ensuring that the language is understandable the first time it is read or heard will improve the quality of education for orthopedic patients undergoing elective hip and knee replacement. Different education techniques and media, as described below, may also increase material absorption and minimize patient overload.

Family/Caregiver Preparedness

Social support is critical for recovery after arthroplasty procedures. In hospitals, arthroplasty patients with strong social support had shorter LOS and were more likely to be discharged home [52]. Commonly, social reasons may be a major factor in why patients are unable to achieve a planned same-day discharge [53]. Previous studies have clearly demonstrated a strong link between patient outcomes and a patient's social support system. The quality of a patient's support system is associated with mortality, mental health, stress, and depression [54]. In addition, even perceived social support can be an important factor after hip or knee replacement [55]. Inadequate caregiver support impacts negatively the quality and rate of recovery after a major operation, regardless of postoperative complications 56.

Some programs may have the patient choose a coach, who commits to attending preoperative care meetings and staying with the patient for a defined period of time following surgery [56]. A family member or caregiver should be present during the preoperative education classes to better prepare for the upcoming surgery. The use of a family member/caregiver, referred to as a "coach," is a critical aspect of successful outcomes after surgery [52, 57]. Some programs make patient and caregiver attendance mandatory and reschedule surgery until the preoperative education class is completed. Others have patients sign contracts that define the social network supporting the patient and outlining the desired postoperative care algorithm in case of complication or readmission. Some programs have a care coordinator do a home visit to make sure that the patient will be able to recover adequately at home under the supervision of a competent caregiver [57]. Regardless of the strategy selected, patients with consistent social support have shorter hospital stays are more likely to be discharged home, more likely to meet ambulation and transfer-out-of-bed targets, score hospital quality of care higher, and are more confident and ready to go home on discharge [52]. The education class provides an opportunity to identify recent changes in the patient's social/family support system, an inability to obtain needed durable medical equipment, failed arrangements for transportation to outpatient physical therapy, unrealistic expectation of discharge to a rehabilitation hospital, and/or other issues that may hinder timely discharge. In this manner, the preoperative class can act as a fail-safe check to make sure patients are appropriately prepared for discharge directly home. Rarely, a patient has no social support. In these circumstances, the problem can be identified in class and the need for a coach can be stressed or discharge plans can be altered.

Evolution of Education Techniques

Traditional education classes combine written handouts with verbal lessons. Learning by at least two different methods can often enhance learning by improving retention and maximizing repetition. Repetition is an effective teaching tool, and using different formats further ensures information retention while avoiding the monotony of single format repetition. The use of animation, video, live demonstrations, and interactive learning are especially helpful in the most successful programs. For example, videos have been shown an effective way to educate [58]. However, video education, like other multimedia techniques, is even more effective when combined with live teaching from a healthcare provider. This may be because, in general, learning via an interactive format is also more successful in accomplishing education goals [59]. Having the education class available on the web for later review can also be useful [60]. Interactive technologies such as virtual reality or web-based learning modules in the comfort of their own home can also teach patients in ways that were not previously possible. These advanced teaching techniques are more engaging for patients and allow a different, and deeper, understanding of the material.

Commonly with elective TJA, group teaching is applicable and has been shown to be very effective. Advantages of group teaching include the benefit of hearing answers to questions from the other participants, group support, and modeling of behavior and skills by the group. The majority of patients responding to a survey after attending a preoperative class preferred verbal education, stating that this was clear and easy to understand [46]. Preoperative education classes for elective TJA have been shown to promote a sense of social connectedness while also fostering participants' independence [43].

Interestingly, many outpatient programs do not offer live joint education camps. Because these cases are shifted away from the hospital setting, a central location for education is often lacking, as is the personnel to teach the classes. Hospitals may be unwilling to provide the staff, space, and resources required to support a joint class if the cases are going to be performed at a freestanding ASC. For this reason, various technologies have become available to fill this void.

A gap between earlier outpatient discharge and first follow-up forms as a consequence of rapid recovery total joint discharges. To fill this void, a significant amount of resources may be required to answer additional phone calls or address questions. Increased personnel to address these questions can be expensive and time-consuming. As a consequence, web-based applications, wearable sensors, mobile apps, virtual follow-ups, and remote care centers have become popular options to assist in monitoring outpatient joint replacement patients. Increased use of technology on the "back-end" of early patient discharges may help minimize complications and readmissions. However, the additional preoperative education on the "front-end" is likely to prepare patients to bridge the outpatient gap and reduce the need for postoperative "touches."

Conclusion

Preoperative education remains a mainstay in the success of total joint replacement programs. The challenges to achieving success in both the bundled payment arena and the transition to outpatient total joints can be addressed through modifications to existing successful preoperative programs. More in-depth focus, with an emphasis on the early expectations for the first few hours at home after outpatient surgery, can improve the probability of postoperative success. In both of the scenarios described, optimizing patient outcomes while minimizing costs is an attainable goal with enhanced preoperative education and preparation.

References

1. Padilla JA, Gabor JA, Kalkut GE, Pazand L, Zuckerman JD, Macaulay W, Bosco JA, Slover JD. Comparison of payment margins between the bundled payments for care improvement initiative and the comprehensive care for joint replacement model Shows a marked reduction for

a successful program. J Bone Joint Surg Am. 2019;101(21):1948–54. https://doi.org/10.2106/JBJS.19.00238.
2. Dobson A, DaVanzo J, Heath S, et al. Medicare payment bundling: insights from claims data and policy implications: analyses of episode-based payment. American Hospital Association and Association of American Medical Colleges; 2012.
3. Miller DC, Gust C, Dimick JB, et al. Large variations in Medicare payments for surgery highlight savings potential from bundled payment programs. Health Aff (Millwood). 2011;30(11):2107. https://doi.org/10.1377/hlthaff.2011.0783.
4. Keswani A, Tasi MC, Fields A, Lovy AJ, Moucha CS, Bozic KJ. Discharge destination after Total joint arthroplasty: an analysis of Postdischarge outcomes, placement risk factors, and recent trends. J Arthroplast. 2016 Jun;31(6):1155–62.
5. Owens JM, Callaghan JJ, Duchman KR, Bedard NA, Otero JE. Short-term morbidity and readmissions increase with skilled nursing facility discharge after Total joint arthroplasty in a Medicare-eligible and skilled nursing facility-eligible patient cohort. J Arthroplast. 2018 May;33(5):1343–7.
6. Ramos NL, Karia RJ, Hutzler LH, et al. The effect of discharge disposition on 30-day readmission rates after total joint arthroplasty. J Arthroplast. 2014;29(4):674. https://doi.org/10.1016/j.arth.2013.09.010.
7. Edwards PK, Mears SC, Barnes CL. BPCI: everyone wins, including the patient. J Arthroplasty. 2017;32(6):1728–31. https://doi.org/10.1016/j.arth.2017.02.014.
8. Luzzi AJ, Fleischman AN, Matthews CN, Crizer MP, Wilsman J, Parvizi J. The "Bundle Busters": incidence and costs of postacute complications following total joint arthroplasty. J Arthroplast. 2018 Sep;33(9):2734–9.
9. Jones S, Alnaib M, Kokkinakis M, Wilkinson M, St Clair Gibson A, Kader D. Pre-operative patient education reduces length of stay after knee joint arthroplasty. Ann R Coll Surg Engl. 2011;93:71–5. https://doi.org/10.1308/003588410X12771863936765.
10. Tait MA, Dredge C, Barnes CL. Preoperative patient education for hip and knee arthroplasty: financial benefit? J Surg Orthop Adv. 2015;24(4):246–51.
11. Edwards PK, Levine M, Cullinan K, Newbern G, Barnes CL. Avoiding readmissions-support systems required after discharge to continue rapid recovery? J Arthroplast. 2015;30(4):527–30. https://doi.org/10.1016/j.arth.2014.12.029.
12. Iorio R, Bosco J, Slover J, Sayeed Y, Zuckerman JD. Single institution early experience with the bundled payments for care improvement initiative. J Bone Joint Surg Am. 2017;99(1):e2. https://doi.org/10.2106/JBJS.16.00066.
13. Pennington JM, Jones DPG, McIntyre S. Clinical pathways in total knee arthroplasty. A New Zealand experience. J Orthop Surg. 2003;11:165–73. https://doi.org/10.1177/230949900301100211.
14. Crowe J, Henderson J. Pre-arthroplasty rehabilitation is effective in reducing hospital stay. Can J Occup Ther. 2003;70:88–96. https://doi.org/10.1177/000841740307000204.
15. Daltroy LH, Morlino CI, Eaton HM, Poss R, Liang MH. Preoperative education for total hip and knee replacement patients. Arthritis Care Res. 1998;11:469–78. https://doi.org/10.1002/art.1790110607.
16. Sjoling M, Nordahl G, Olofsson N, Asplund K. The impact of pre-operative information on state anxiety, postoperative pain and satisfaction with pain management. Patient Educ Couns. 2003;51:169–76. https://doi.org/10.1016/S0738-3991(02)00191-X.
17. Giraudet-Le Quintrec JS, Coste J, Vastel L, Pacault V, Jeanne L, Lamas JP, et al. Positive effect of patient education for hip surgery: a randomized trial. Clin Orthop Relat R. 2003;1:112–20. https://doi.org/10.1097/01.blo.0000079268.91782.bc.
18. Gammon J, Mulholland CW. Effect of preparatory information prior to elective total hip replacement on post-operative physical coping outcomes. Int J Nurs Stud. 1996;33:589–604. https://doi.org/10.1016/S0020-7489(96)00019-3.

19. Moulton LS, Evans PA, Starks I, Smith T. Pre-operative education prior to elective hip arthroplasty surgery improves postoperative outcome. Int Orthop. 2015;39(8):1483–6. https://doi.org/10.1007/s00264-015-2754-2.
20. Feng JE, Novikov D, Anoushiravani AA, Schwarzkopf R. Total knee arthroplasty: improving outcomes with a multidisciplinary approach. J Multidiscip Healthc. 2018;11:63–73.
21. Spalding NJ. Reducing anxiety by pre-operative education: make the future familiar. Occup Ther Int. 2003;10:278–93. https://doi.org/10.1002/oti.191.
22. Jahic D, Omerovic D, Tanovic AT, Dzankovic F, Campara MT. The effect of prehabilitation on postoperative outcome in patients following primary total knee arthroplasty. Mediev Archaeol. 2018;72(6):439–43. https://doi.org/10.5455/medarh.2018.72.439-443.
23. Clode-Baker E, Draper E, Raymond N, Haslam C, Gregg P. Preparing patients for total hip replacement: a randomized controlled trial of preoperative education intervention. J Health Psychol. 1997;2:107–14. https://doi.org/10.1177/135910539700200111.
24. Claeys M, Mosher C, Reesman D. The POP program: the patient education advantage. Orthop Nurs. 1998;17(4):37–47. https://doi.org/10.1097/00006416-199807000-00008.
25. Jahic D, Omerovic D, Tanovic AT, Dzankovic F, Dorr LD CMT, Chao L. The emotional state of the patient after total hip and knee arthroplasty. Clin Orthop Relat Res. 2007;463:7–12.
26. Lin PC, Lin LC, Lin JJ. Comparing the effectiveness of different educational programs for patients with total knee arthroplasty. Orthop Nurs. 1997;16:43–9. https://doi.org/10.1097/00006416-199709000-00013.
27. Sisak K, Darch R, Burgess LC, Middleton RG, Wainwright TW. A preoperative education class reduces length of stay for total knee replacement patients identified at risk of an extended length of stay. J Rehabil Med. 2019;51(10):788–96. https://doi.org/10.2340/16501977-2602.
28. Pelt CE, Gililland JM, Erickson JA, Trimble DE, Anderson MB, Peters CL. Improving value in total joint arthroplasty: a comprehensive patient education and management program decreases discharge to post-acute care facilities and post-operative complications. J Arthroplast. 2018 Jan;33(1):14–8.
29. Edwards PK, Mears SC, Barnes CL. Preoperative education for hip and knee replacement: never stop learning. Curr Rev Musculoskelet Med. 2017;10(3):356–64.
30. Majid N, Lee S, Plummer V. The effectiveness of orthopedic patient education in improving patient outcomes: a systematic review protocol. JBI Database System Rev Implement Rep. 2015 Jan;13(1):122–33.
31. Sah A. Considerations for office and staff protocols for outpatient joint replacement. J Arthroplast. 2019;34(7):S44–5.
32. Churchill L, Pollock M, Lebedeva Y, Pasic N, Bryant D, Howard J, Lanting B, Laliberte Rudman D. Optimizing outpatient total hip arthroplasty: perspectives of key stakeholders. Can J Surg. 2018;61(6):370–6. https://doi.org/10.1503/cjs.016117.
33. Mancuso CA, Graziano S, Briskie LM, Peterson MG, Pellicci PM, Salvati EA, Sculco TP. Randomized trials to modify patients' preoperative expectations of hip and knee arthroplasties. Clin Orthop Relat Res. 2008;466:424–31. https://doi.org/10.1007/s11999-007-0052-z.
34. Loft M, McWilliam C, Ward-Griffin C. Patient empowerment after total hip and knee replacement. Orthop Nurs. 2003;22:42–7. https://doi.org/10.1097/00006416-200301000-00012.
35. Lucas B. Preparing patients for hip and knee surgery. Nurs Stand. 2007;22:50–8. https://doi.org/10.7748/ns2007.09.22.2.50.c4618.
36. Tilbury C, Haanstra TM, Leichtenberg CS, Verdegaal SH, Ostelo RW, de Vet HC, Nelissen RG, Vliet Vlieland TP. Unfulfilled expectations after total hip and knee arthroplasty surgery: there is a need for better preoperative patient information and education. J Arthroplast. 2016;31(10):2139–45. https://doi.org/10.1016/j.arth.2016.02.061.
37. Scott CE, Bugler KE, Clement ND, MacDonald D, Howie CR, Biant LC. Patient expectations of arthroplasty of the hip and knee. J Bone Joint Surg (Br). 2012;94:974–81. https://doi.org/10.1302/0301-620X.94B7.28219.Graziano.
38. Ghomrawi HMK, Lee LY, Nwachukwu BU, Jain D, Wright T, Padgett D, Bozic KJ, Lyman S. Preoperative expectations associated with postoperative dissatisfaction after total knee

arthroplasty: a cohort study. J Am Acad Orthop Surg. 2020;28(4):e145–50. https://doi.org/10.5435/JAAOS-D-18-00785.
39. Nilsdotter AK, Toksvig-Larsen S, Roos EM. Knee arthroplasty: are patients' expectations fulfilled? A prospective study of pain and function in 102 patients with 5-year follow-up. Acta Orthop. 2009;80(1):55–61. https://doi.org/10.1080/17453670902805007.
40. Ghomrawi HM, Franco Ferrando N, Mandl LA, Do H, Noor N, Gonzalez Della Valle A. How often are patient and surgeon recovery expectations for total joint arthroplasty aligned? Results of a pilot study. HSS J. 2011;7:229–34. https://doi.org/10.1007/s11420-011-9203-6.
41. Zietek P, Zarzycka B, Zietek J, Stepien-Slodkowska M, Sienko-Awierianow E, Kotrych D, Dobiecki K. The impact of caregivers' anxiety on patients' anxiety before fast-track knee arthroplasty. Acta Chir Orthop Traumatol Cechoslov. 2017;84(4):292–8.
42. Brander Victoria A, David SS, Adams Angela D, Norman HR, Stephen B, Stanos Steven P, Timothy H. Predicting total knee replacement pain: a prospective, observational study. Clin Orthop Relat Res. 2003;416:27–36. https://doi.org/10.1097/01.blo.0000092983.12414.e9.
43. Lane-Carlson ML, Kumar J. Engaging patients in managing their health care: patient perceptions of the effect of a total joint replacement presurgical class. Perm J. 2012;16(3):42–7.
44. Medina-Garzón M. Effectiveness of a nursing intervention to diminish preoperative anxiety in patients programmed for knee replacement surgery: preventive controlled and randomized clinical trial. Investig Educ Enferm. 2019;37(2):e07. https://doi.org/10.17533/udea.iee.v37n2e07.
45. Riddle Daniel L, Wade James B, Jiranek WA, Xiangrong K. Preoperative pain catastrophizing predicts pain outcome after knee arthroplasty. Clin Orthop Relat Res. 2010;468(3):798–806. https://doi.org/10.1007/s11999-009-0963-y.
46. Chetty C, Ehlers VJ. Orthopaedic patients' perceptions about their pre-operative information. Curationis. 2009;32(4):55–60. https://doi.org/10.4102/curationis.v32i4.992.
47. Brander V, Gondek S, Martin E, Stulberg SD. THE JOHN INSALL AWARD: pain and depression influence outcome 5 years after knee replacement surgery. Clin Orthop Relat Res. 2007;464:21–6.
48. Tong F, Dannaway J, Enke O, Eslick G. Effect of preoperative psychological interventions on elective orthopaedic surgery outcomes: a systematic review and meta-analysis. ANZ J Surg. 2020;90(3):230–6. https://doi.org/10.1111/ans.15332.
49. Kudibal MT, Kallemose T, Troelsen A, Husted H, Gromov K. Does ethnicity and education influence preoperative disability and expectations in patients undergoing total knee arthroplasty? World J Orthop. 2018;9(10):220–8. https://doi.org/10.5312/wjo.v9.i10.220.
50. Baker DW, Parker RM, Williams MV, Clark WS, Nurss J. The relationship of patient reading ability to self-reported health and use of health services. Am J Public Health. 1997;87:1027–30. https://doi.org/10.2105/AJPH.87.6.1027.
51. Hadden KB, Prince LY, Bushmiaer MK, Watson JC, Barnes CL. Health literacy and surgery expectations in total hip and knee arthroplasty patients. Patient Educ Couns. 2018;101(10):1823–7. https://doi.org/10.1016/j.pec.2018.05.021.
52. Theiss MM, Ellison MW, Tea CG, Warner JF, Silver RM, Murphy VJ. The connection between strong social support and joint replacement outcomes. Orthopedics. 2011;34(5):357.
53. Cody JP, Pfefferle KJ, Ammeen DJ, Fricka KB. Is outpatient unicompartmental knee arthroplasty safe to perform at an ambulatory surgery center? A comparative study of early post-operative complications. J Arthroplast. 2018;33:673–6.
54. Mitchinson AR, Kim HM, Geisser M, Rosenberg JM, Hinshaw DB. Social connectedness and patient recovery after major operations. J Am Coll Surg. 2008;206(2):292–300. https://doi.org/10.1016/j.jamcollsurg.2007.08.017.
55. van den Akker-Scheek I, Stevens M, Spriensma A, van Horn JR. Groningen orthopaedic social support scale: validity and reliability. J Adv Nurs. 2004;47(1):57–63. https://doi.org/10.1111/j.1365-2648.2004.03065.x.

56. Parcells BW, Giacobbe D, Macknet D, Smith A, Schottenfeld M, Harwood DA, Kayiaros S. Total joint arthroplasty in a stand-alone ambulatory surgical center: short-term outcomes. Orthopedics. 2016;39:223–8.
57. Bert JM, Hooper J, Moen S. Outpatient total joint arthroplasty. Curr Rev Musculoskelet Med. 2017;10:567–74.
58. Freda MC, Abruzzo M, Davini D, DeVore N, Damus K, Merkatz IR. Are they watching? Are they learning? Prenatal video education in the waiting room. J Perinat Ed. 1994;3:20–8.
59. Herrmann KS, Kreuzer H. A randomized prospective study on anxiety reduction by preparatory disclosure with and without video film show about a planned heart catheterization. Eur Heart J. 1989;10(8):753–7. https://doi.org/10.1093/oxfordjournals.eurheartj.a059560.
60. O'Connor MI, Brennan K, Kazmerchak S, Pratt J. YouTube videos to create a "virtual hospital experience" for hip and knee replacement patients to decrease preoperative anxiety: a randomized trial. Interact J Med Res. 2016;5(2):e10. https://doi.org/10.2196/ijmr.4295.

Chapter 5
Multimodal Pain Management Protocols for THA and TKA

Elizabeth B. Gausden, Mark W. Pagnano, and Matthew P. Abdel

Introduction

Improved perioperative pain control made possible through advances in multimodal pain management may be the single most important factor that has facilitated outpatient total joint arthroplasty (TJA). Inadequate pain control following total hip arthroplasty (THA) or total knee arthroplasty (TKA) is associated with longer hospital stays, readmissions, lower patient satisfaction, as well as decreased knee range of motion for TKA patients [1]. Multimodal analgesia (MMA) has emerged as the gold standard for patients following THAs and TKAs. This strategy enlists multiple analgesics with varying mechanisms of action in order to produce a synergistic effect of pain relief. In addition to lowering the amount of opioids required for similar levels of pain relief, multiple studies have demonstrated that the use of MMA is associated with improved patient outcome and satisfaction, reduced hospital stays, and lower resource utilization [2, 3]. Pain can be separated broadly into emanating from both the neurogenic and inflammatory pathways, and the goal of MMA is to block all possible pain pathways. Oral analgesia, regional anesthesia, peripheral nerve blocks (PNBs), and parental analgesia are all components of MMA. Furthermore, MMA can be categorized temporally, starting with preoperative dosing of oral or parenteral analgesia, intraoperative use of regional anesthesia, parenteral analgesia and periarticular infiltration of analgesia, and finally postoperative analgesia in the post-anesthesia care unit, during floor care, and at home.

E. B. Gausden · M. W. Pagnano · M. P. Abdel (✉)
Department of Orthopedic Surgery, Mayo Clinic, Rochester, MN, USA
e-mail: Gausden.elizabeth@mayo.edu; Pagnano.mark@mayo.edu; Abdel.matthew@mayo.edu

R. M. Meneghini, L. T. Buller (eds.), *Outpatient Hip and Knee Replacement*,
https://doi.org/10.1007/978-3-031-27037-6_5

Anti-Inflammatories and Acetaminophen

Prostaglandins are synthesized by local tissues during TJA, triggering an inflammatory pain cascade. Preoperative administration of nonsteroidal anti-inflammatory drugs (NSAIDs) theoretically reduces the early production of prostaglandins in tissues during TJAs and reduces pain postoperatively. Multiple randomized clinical trials (RCTs) have proven the efficacy of this technique of preoperative NSAID administration to reduce postoperative opioid use, as well as pain, vomiting, sleep disturbance, and improve knee range of motion in TKA patients [4, 5]. Theoretically, preemptive analgesia prevents sensitization of pain receptors in the peripheral and central nervous systems as once these sensors are triggered initially, a lower pain threshold is required for triggering them in the postoperative period [6]. The potential downside of using NSAIDs prior to surgery is an increased risk of bleeding intraoperatively and postoperatively, but this theoretical risk has not been borne out in studies. Continuation of NSAIDs for 2 weeks following TJA is recommended as they will continue to attenuate the production of prostaglandins, mediating the pain experienced and do not require tapering for discontinuation.

Cyclooxygenase-2 (COX-2) inhibitors offer the benefit of selective inhibition of COX-2 receptors that are increased in inflammation while sparing the constitutively expressed COX-1 receptors regulate platelet function and line gastrointestinal mucosa. As a result, the use of COX-2 inhibitors results in fewer adverse effects compared to nonselective NSAIDs, such as diclofenac, ibuprofen, or naproxen, including less GI complaints and platelet dysfunction. Buvanendran et al. [4] performed an RCT to study the efficacy of perioperative rofecoxib, a COX-2 inhibitor, versus placebo in patients undergoing TKA and found that the COX-2 inhibitor reduced overall opioid consumption, pain, vomiting, sleep disturbance, and improved knee range of motion.

Acetaminophen also reduces the production of prostaglandins, but via a poorly understood mechanism independent of that of NSAIDs. Nevertheless, the combination of acetaminophen and NSAIDs reduces the amount of opioids consumed by TJA patients compared to the administration of NSAIDs alone [7–9]. The use of oral acetaminophen may be as effective as intravenous (IV) acetaminophen in terms of improving analgesia in postoperative TJA patients [10]. Using a dose of 1000 mg of acetaminophen compared to 650 mg has demonstrated superiority in pain relief [11, 12], and that is incorporated into our institution's MMA protocol (Table 5.1).

Table 5.1 Mayo multimodal opioid-sparing pain protocol [50]

Preoperative	Details and Dosing
Acetaminophen	1000 mg PO followed by q6h IV dosing in the OR
Celecoxib	400 mg PO once
Caffeine	200 mg PO if the patient consumes >100 mg of caffeine daily
Peripheral nerve blockade	
Single shot Adductor Canal block/ saphenous nerve block for TKA	10 mL of 0.5% bupivacaine 1:200,000 epinephrine ± 50 μg dexmedetomidine
Lumbar plexus block/psoas nerve catheter	Complex revision hips, surgeon preference
Femoral nerve catheter	Revision knees, chronic pain, surgeon preference
Adductor canal catheter	Chronic pain/opioid tolerance, surgeon preference
Intraoperative care	
Single-shot spinal	Intermediate-acting mepivacaine or low-dose bupivacaine spinal without long-acting opioid
Sedation	Propofol infusion titrated to effect
Periarticular injection (PAI)	**According to surgeon preference**
Antiemetics	Ondansetron 4 mg IV, dexamethasone 0.1 mg/kg up to 8 mg
Ketamine	10–40 mg IV divided doses through perioperative period (10 mg IV/h recommended)
Post-anesthesia care unit (PACU)	
Acetaminophen	1000 mg PO or IV once for pain
Oxycodone	5–10 mg PO q4 h PRN pain (5 mg for pain level 4–6; 10 mg for pain level > 6)
Hydromorphone	2–4 mg PO q4 h for pain in patients with allergies or intolerance to oxycodone
Floor care	
Acetaminophen	1000 mg PO q6 h
Ketorolac	15 mg IV q6 h for 4 doses (if GFR >50 mL/min)
Celecoxib	200 mg PO BID starting after 4 doses of ketorolac (only if GFR >50 mL/min)
Dexamethasone	8 mg IV once on POD1 morning for patients <65 years old; 4 mg IV once on POD1 morning for patients 66–80-years old
Tramadol	50–100 mg PO q4 h PRN pain (use 50 mg for pain rated 3; use 100 mg for pain rated 4 or greater)
Oxycodone	5–10 mg PO q4 h PRN pain (5 for pain rated 4–6; 10 mg for pain rated 7–10)
Fentanyl	25 μg IV q15 min PRN for pain 7–10 for 3 doses
Hydromorphone	0.2 mg IV q15 min PRN for pain 7–10 for 3 doses (for those with intolerance to fentanyl)

Gabapentinoids

Pregabalin and gabapentin are gamma-aminobutyric acid (GABA) receptor inhibitors that desensitize pain pathways in the central nervous system. Gabapentin specifically acts on presynaptic voltage-gated calcium channels that are upregulated in nerve injury and decreases the hyperexcitability of secondary nociceptive neurons in the dorsal horn of the spinal cord. Gabapentin was originally marketed in 1993 as an antiepileptic, and since then has been used to treat neuropathic pain. While not specifically approved by the Food and Drug Administration (FDA) for perioperative pain control, there is evidence that the use of gabapentinoids in THA and TKA patients may decrease opioid usage. Zhai et al. [13] completed a meta-analysis examining the effect of gabapentin on acute postoperative pain in TKA patients. Their study included 769 patients and concluded that gabapentin results in superior pain relief compared to a placebo for pain control after TKA.

Similarly, a meta-analysis of studies using pregabalin in TKA concluded that pregabalin reduced cumulative morphine consumption at 24 and 48 h postoperatively, and improved postoperative knee flexion at 48 h compared to patients treated with placebo [14].

A concerning association between gabapentin use and respiratory depression, as well as naloxone administration, has been identified recently [15, 16]. Similarly, concomitant use of gabapentin in opioid users was associated with a 49% increased risk of death from an opioid overdose in a case-control study of over 5000 patients [17]. This association could be related to the additive effects of both drugs on suppressing respiratory drive or increased absorption of gabapentin in the setting of opioid use [17]. For these reasons, we have begun to discourage gabapentinoids as part of MMA at our institution.

Steroids

The antiemetic and anti-inflammatory effects of steroids are well demonstrated in the perioperative setting [18, 19]. In an RCT, Backes et al. [20] studied the effect of 10 mg of intravenous dexamethasone administered intraoperatively to patients undergoing TJA and found that those treated with the steroid consumed less rescue antiemetic and analgesic medications, and reported less pain and nausea. Those treated with the IV steroid also had a significantly shorter length of stay and ambulated further distances compared to the control group [20]. Potential risks associated with perioperative steroid administration include poor glucose control, theoretically increased infection risk, and gastrointestinal hemorrhage and need to be weighed against the potential benefits in each TJA patient. We generally use dexamethasone IV intraoperatively and administer an additional dose the morning after TJA for patients under 80-years old (Table 5.1). Dexamethasone in intermediate doses or higher, approximately 8–10 mg, can have a positive analgesic effect as well, and pain is improved when steroids are administered in the first 48 h after surgery [21].

Opioids

Opioid receptors, found predominantly in the central nervous system, peripheral nervous system, and gastrointestinal tract, mediate the physical and psychoactive experience of pain. Previously, opioid administration in the perioperative setting was done through patient-controlled analgesia (PCA) devices that allowed IV administration of opioids in response to patients pushing a button. PCA usage is in steady decline in the past decade as evidence has emerged illustrating the superiority of multimodal approaches [22, 23].

A thorough evaluation of a patient's use of opioids is fundamental to planning a perioperative pain regimen. Sing et al. [24] found that patients using opioids preoperatively required more than 50 mean milligram of morphine equivalents over the course of their hospital stay compared to patients who were non-opioid users preoperatively. Weaning patients from opioids preoperatively may be an effective strategy to lower the incidence of perioperative complications, as Jain et al. [25] identified lower complication rates in patients who had stopped using opioids within 3 months of surgery. If weaning opioids is not possible, then selective use of PCAs for patients with preoperative opioid dependence may be warranted. Further, if patients are opioid dependent preoperatively, they may not be a candidate for same-day discharge in the outpatient setting unless they are capable of weaning off the narcotics prior to surgery, or there is a detailed plan to assist with their pain control at home postoperatively.

Prescribing habits for postoperative opioids to be taken upon discharge home have also changed as a result of greater awareness of the opioid epidemic. Huang et al. [26] compared opioid usage postoperatively between THA and TKA patients and identified higher consumption of pain pills in TKA patients (37 pills was the median for THA patients and 67 pills for TKA patients), and TKA patients were five times more likely to ask for a refill compared to THA patients. Hannon et al. [27] revealed the median number of unused pills was 15 for patients who were given a prescription for 30 tablets of 5 mg oxycodone immediate release (IR) compared to 73 unused pills for those patients given 90 tablets following TJA, with no difference in pain scores or patient-reported outcome scores at 6 weeks postoperatively. From our institution, Wyles et al. [23] demonstrated the efficacy of implementing institutional guidelines (in this case a limit of 400 oral morphine equivalents which is comparable to 50 tablets of 5 mg oxycodone) for reducing opioid prescription in arthroplasty patients.

Neuraxial Anesthesia

Multiple studies have indicated the superiority of neuraxial anesthesia compared to general endotracheal anesthesia (GETA) for patients undergoing THA or TKA [28, 29]. Advantages of neuraxial anesthesia for TJA patients include decreased risk of surgical site infection, shorter surgical time, lower rates of deep vein thromboses and pulmonary emboli, lower risk of pulmonary complications, less intraoperative bleeding, lower transfusion rates, and lower length of hospital stay [28–31]. Despite the documented benefits, the risks of neuraxial anesthesia include spinal hematoma, epidural abscess, and nerve injury, and these risks must be weighed against the benefits for every individual patient, especially those requiring chronic anticoagulation [32].

Neuraxial anesthesia includes spinal and epidural anesthesia and the combination of the two techniques. Weinstein et al. [33] compared combined spinal epidural (CSE) anesthesia, spinal anesthesia, and epidural anesthesia in patients undergoing THA and TKA and concluded that a single-shot spinal technique resulted in reduced odds for cardiac, pulmonary, gastrointestinal, and thromboembolic events. The authors suggest that spinal anesthesia resulted in a more complete block during surgery, resulting in less pain.

Unpublished data from a study recently completed at our institution, including two of the coauthors of this chapter (MWP and MPA), compared spinal anesthesia with an intermediate-acting local anesthetic, mepivacaine, to the more traditional longer acting bupivacaine [34]. We found that spinal anesthesia using mepivacaine allowed for a faster return of lower extremity function compared to bupivacaine (185 min compared to 214 min, $p = 0.01$). Therefore, mepivacaine may be a better agent for the outpatient setting and same-day discharge of THA and TKA patients.

Peripheral Nerve Blocks

Peripheral nerve blocks (PNB) following THA and TKA can provide longer acting anesthesia for patients and act as a major contributor to limiting opioid usage as part of MMA [35]. There are a variety of PNBs currently used as one modality of pain control for THA and TKA, including posterior lumbar plexus nerve block ("psoas block"), femoral nerve block (FNB), interspace between the popliteal artery and posterior capsule of the knee (iPACK), sciatic nerve block (SCB), adductor canal block (ACB), and fascia iliaca block. Like any modality, the benefit of PNBs must be weighed against their potential risks, which include increased risk of falls and delayed progress with ambulation secondary to motor blockade, peripheral nerve injury, and prolonged dysesthesias. Ilfeld et al. [36] reported a 7% risk of a postoperative fall in patients who received a FNB or lumbar plexus block.

The ACB is more distal than a typical femoral nerve block, which allows for the preservation of quadriceps function and facilitates early ambulation [37]. For this reason, at our institution, we prefer a single-shot adductor canal block/saphenous nerve block for most primary TKAs in order to achieve the benefit of the sensory blockade and pain relief while maintaining motor function for same-day ambulation.

Continuous indwelling catheters left to provide sustained nerve blocks throughout the postoperative period have also been studied in arthroplasty patients. Spangehl et al. [38] compared three regimens in primary TKA patients: the first a continuous femoral nerve catheter, the second a single-shot SCB, and the third a PAI cocktail of ropivacaine, ketorolac, epinephrine, and morphine. There were no differences between patients who had the single-shot SCB compared to those with the indwelling femoral nerve catheter, but both of the block groups had more falls, lower quadriceps function on postoperative day 1, and more peripheral nerve dysesthesias at 6 weeks postoperatively. Similarly, Elkassabany et al. [39] completed an RCT comparing a single-shot ACB to a continuous ACB in TKA, finding no difference between groups in terms of opioid consumption, length of hospital stay, or functional outcomes. Amundson et al. [40] compared TKA patients treated with either a femoral nerve catheter plus sciatic nerve blocks, ropivacaine-based PAI, or liposomal bupivacaine-based PAI in an RCT and found that the PAI groups were comparable to the femoral nerve catheter with sciatic nerve block group in terms of maximal pain scores on postoperative days 1 and 2. At our institution, indwelling catheter nerve blocks are reserved for revisions or exceptional cases of patients with preoperative chronic pain (Table 5.1).

In THA patients, various studies have concluded that the use of PNBs does not result in superior pain control or lower opioid consumption. Nielsen et al. [41] studied obturator nerve blocks (ONBs) in a RCT of THA patients also undergoing spinal anesthesia, finding equivalent opioid consumption and no difference in the level of pain or nausea compared to a placebo. In an RCT from our institution, Johnson et al. [42] compared continuous lumbar plexus block to periarticular injection (PAI) in THA and found no substantial difference in terms of maximal pain or opioid consumption postoperatively. Similarly, a recent meta-analysis including 2296 patients demonstrated no difference between local infiltration analgesia and PNBs in terms of analgesia or opioid consumption 24 h after THA. For this reason, our institutional protocol for THA is a single-shot spinal anesthetic with PAI at the time of surgery including ketorolac, morphine, bupivacaine, and a steroid. We selectively use lumbar plexus blocks for complex revision hips and according to specific surgeon preferences (Table 5.1).

Periarticular Injections (Pais)

In the early 2000s, surgeons and anesthesiologists began using PAIs in THAs and TKAS. These PAIs typically consist of various combinations of long and short-acting local anesthetics, nonsteroidal anti-inflammatories, opioids, and adjuncts such as epinephrine. There is an abundance of evidence demonstrating the efficacy of PAIs in reducing postoperative pain levels, and opioid usage [38, 43]. The evidence that PAI is as effective as certain PNBs for patients undergoing arthroplasty is also growing [42, 44]. The optimal dosage and combination of local anesthetic and adjuvants in the PAIs used in THAs and TKAs remains to be determined. Kelley et al. [45] compared two PAI cocktails and found less postoperative pain when ketorolac was included along with local anesthetic and epinephrine in the cocktail.

There is some evidence that administration of the PAI earlier in the surgical procedure (i.e., prior to incising tissues) may be superior to administration of PAI at the late stages of arthroplasty [46]. This could be related to the preemptive block of pain receptors resulting in the prevention of hypersensitization to pain in the postoperative period, similar to the oral administration of anti-inflammatories prior to surgery.

The use of liposomal bupivacaine-based PAIs that allows for delayed delivery of local anesthetic over time has also been proposed. Multiple studies have compared liposomal bupivacaine to conventional bupivacaine when used in PAIs in arthroplasty, and most have found no difference in postoperative pain or opioid consumption [40, 47–49]. Given the increased cost associated with liposomal bupivacaine, we are no longer using this form in PAIs at our institution.

Conclusion

Contemporary multimodal pain management is an essential component of a successful outpatient arthroplasty program and employs anesthetics and analgesics of varying mechanisms of action and via various routes of administration perioperatively to prevent hypersensitization of pain receptors and to target multiple pain pathways. The appropriate use of MMA in arthroplasty patients results in fewer complications, lower opioid consumption, lower cost, and faster return to function. While the ideal combination of anesthetic and analgesic techniques is likely to vary based on individual surgeon and practice variables, it is clear that patients will benefit from a deliberate, coordinated approach to pain management that includes the preoperative, intraoperative, and postoperative periods. Failure to provide a thoughtful MMA program undoubtedly increases the risk of failure to discharge and readmissions when performing same-day discharge outpatient THA and TKA.

References

1. Roberts C, Foster D, Shi GG, Lesser ER, Heckman MG, Whalen JL, et al. A collaborative approach to pain control reduces in-hospital opioid use and improves range of motion following total knee arthroplasty. Cureus. 2019;11(5):e4678. http://www.ncbi.nlm.nih.gov/pubmed/31328069.
2. Duncan CM, Moeschler SM, Horlocker TT, Hanssen AD, Hebl JR. A self-paired comparison of perioperative outcomes before and after implementation of a clinical pathway in patients undergoing total knee arthroplasty. Reg Anesth Pain Med. 2019;38(6):533–8. http://www.ncbi.nlm.nih.gov/pubmed/24121605.
3. Hebl JR, Dilger JA, Byer DE, Kopp SL, Stevens SR, Pagnano MW, et al. A pre-emptive multimodal pathway featuring peripheral nerve block improves perioperative outcomes after major orthopedic surgery. Reg Anesth Pain Med. 2008;33(6):510–7.
4. Buvanendran A, Kroin JS, Tuman KJ, Lubenow TR, Elmofty D, Moric M, et al. Effects of perioperative administration of a selective cyclooxygenase 2 inhibitor on pain management and recovery of function after knee replacement: a randomized controlled trial. JAMA. 2003;290(18):2411–8. http://www.ncbi.nlm.nih.gov/pubmed/14612477.
5. Huang YM, Wang CM, Wang CT, Lin WP, Horng LC, Jiang CC. Perioperative celecoxib administration for pain management after total knee arthroplasty–a randomized, controlled study. BMC Musculoskelet Disord. 2008;9:77. http://www.ncbi.nlm.nih.gov/pubmed/18519002.
6. Moucha CS, Weiser MC, Levin EJ. Current strategies in anesthesia and analgesia for total knee arthroplasty. J Am Acad Orthop Surg. 2016;24:60–73.

7. Thybo KH, Hägi-Pedersen D, Dahl JB, Wetterslev J, Nersesjan M, Jakobsen JC, et al. Effect of combination of paracetamol (acetaminophen) and ibuprofen vs either alone on patient-controlled morphine consumption in the first 24 hours after total hip arthroplasty: the PANSAID randomized clinical trial. JAMA. 2019;321(6):562–71. http://www.ncbi.nlm.nih.gov/pubmed/30747964.
8. Murata-Ooiwa M, Tsukada S, Wakui M. Intravenous acetaminophen in multimodal pain management for patients undergoing total knee arthroplasty: a randomized, double-blind, placebo-controlled trial. J Arthroplast. 2017;32(10):3024–8.
9. Gupta A, Abubaker H, Demas E, Ahrendtsen L. A randomized trial comparing the safety and efficacy of intravenous ibuprofen versus ibuprofen and acetaminophen in knee or hip arthroplasty. Pain Physician. 2016;19(6):349–56.
10. Politi JR, Davis RL, Matrka AK. Randomized prospective trial comparing the use of intravenous versus oral acetaminophen in total joint arthroplasty. J Arthroplast. 2017;32(4):1125–7. http://www.ncbi.nlm.nih.gov/pubmed/27839957.
11. Qi DS, May LG, Zimmerman B, Peng P, Atillasoy E, Brown JD, et al. A randomized, double-blind, placebo-controlled study of acetaminophen 1000 mg versus acetaminophen 650 mg for the treatment of postsurgical dental pain. Clin Ther. 2012;34(12):2247–2258.e3. http://www.ncbi.nlm.nih.gov/pubmed/23200183.
12. Moore RA, Derry S, Wiffen PJ, Straube S, Aldington DJ. Overview review: comparative efficacy of oral ibuprofen and paracetamol (acetaminophen) across acute and chronic pain conditions. Eur J Pain. 2015;19(9):1213–23. http://www.ncbi.nlm.nih.gov/pubmed/25530283.
13. Zhai L, Song Z, Liu K. The effect of gabapentin on acute Postoperative pain in patients undergoing total knee arthroplasty. Medicine (United States). 2016;95:e3673. Lippincott Williams and Wilkins.
14. Han C, Kuang MJ, Ma JX, Ma XL. Is pregabalin effective and safe in total knee arthroplasty? A PRISMA-compliant meta-analysis of randomized-controlled trials. Medicine (Baltimore). 2017;96(26):e6947. http://www.ncbi.nlm.nih.gov/pubmed/28658096.
15. Cavalcante AN, Sprung J, Schroeder DR, Weingarten TN. Multimodal analgesic therapy with gabapentin and its association with postoperative respiratory depression. Anesth Analg. 2017;125(1):141–6. http://www.ncbi.nlm.nih.gov/pubmed/27984223.
16. Deljou A, Hedrick SJ, Portner ER, Schroeder DR, Hooten WM, Sprung J, et al. Pattern of perioperative gabapentinoid use and risk for postoperative naloxone administration. Br J Anaesth. 2018;120(4):798–806.
17. Gomes T, Juurlink DN, Antoniou T, Mamdani MM, Paterson JM, van den Brink W. Gabapentin, opioids, and the risk of opioid-related death: a population-based nested case–control study. PLoS Med. 2017;14(10):e1002396.
18. Cheng BLY, So EHK, Hui GKM, Yung BPK, Tsui ASK, Wang OKF, et al. Pre-operative intravenous steroid improves pain and joint mobility after total knee arthroplasty in Chinese population: a double-blind randomized controlled trial. Eur J Orthop Surg Traumatol. 2019;29:1473.
19. Koh IJ, Chang CB, Lee JH, Jeon YT, Kim TK. Preemptive low-dose dexamethasone reduces postoperative emesis and pain after TKA: a randomized controlled study. Clin Orthop Relat Res. 2013;471(9):3010–20. http://www.ncbi.nlm.nih.gov/pubmed/23645340.
20. Backes JR, Bentley JC, Politi JR, Chambers BT. Dexamethasone reduces length of hospitalization and improves postoperative pain and nausea after total joint arthroplasty: a prospective, randomized controlled trial. J Arthroplast. 2013;28(8 SUPPL):11–7.
21. Fan ZR, Ma J, Ma XL, Wang Y, Sun L, Wang Y, et al. The efficacy of dexamethasone on pain and recovery after total hip arthroplasty. Medicine (Baltimore). 2018;97:e0100. Lippincott Williams and Wilkins.
22. Chen PY, Samy W, Aaron Ying CL. Comparing cost and effectiveness of IVPCA morphine with perioperative multimodal analgesia of oral etoricoxib and oxycontin: a retrospective study. J Orthop. 2019;16(6):585–9. http://www.ncbi.nlm.nih.gov/pubmed/31660027.
23. Wyles CC, Hevesi M, Trousdale ER, Ubl DS, Gazelka HM, Habermann EB, et al. The 2018 Chitranjan S. Ranawat, MD award: developing and implementing a novel institutional guide-

line strategy reduced postoperative opioid prescribing after TKA and THA. Clin Orthop Relat Res. 2019;477(1):104–13. http://www.ncbi.nlm.nih.gov/pubmed/30794233.
24. Sing DC, Barry JJ, Cheah JW, Vail TP, Hansen EN. Long-acting opioid use independently predicts perioperative complication in total joint arthroplasty. J Arthroplast. 2016;31(9 Suppl):170–174.e1. http://www.ncbi.nlm.nih.gov/pubmed/27451080.
25. Jain N, Brock JL, Malik AT, Phillips FM, Khan SN. Prediction of complications, readmission, and revision surgery based on duration of preoperative opioid use: analysis of major joint replacement and lumbar fusion. J Bone Joint Surg Am. 2019;101(5):384–91. http://www.ncbi.nlm.nih.gov/pubmed/30845032.
26. Huang PS, Copp SN. Oral opioids are overprescribed in the opiate-naive patient undergoing total joint arthroplasty. J Am Acad Orthop Surg. 2019;27(15):e702–8. http://www.ncbi.nlm.nih.gov/pubmed/30676515.
27. Hannon CP, Calkins TE, Li J, Culvern C, Darrith B, Nam D, et al. The James A. Rand Young investigator's award: large opioid prescriptions are unnecessary after total joint arthroplasty: a randomized controlled trial. J Arthroplast. 2019;34(7S):S4–10. http://www.ncbi.nlm.nih.gov/pubmed/30799266
28. Pugely AJ, Martin CT, Gao Y, Mendoza-Lattes S, Callaghan JJ. Differences in short-term complications between spinal and general anesthesia for primary total knee arthroplasty. J Bone Joint Surg Am. 2013;95(3):193–9.
29. Basques BA, Toy JO, Bohl DD, Golinvaux NS, Grauer JN. General compared with spinal anesthesia for total hip arthroplasty. J Bone Joint Surg Am. 2015;97(6):455–61.
30. Helwani MA, Avidan MS, Ben Abdallah A, Kaiser DJ, Clohisy JC, Hall BL, et al. Effects of regional versus general anesthesia on outcomes after total hip arthroplasty: a retrospective propensity-matched cohort study. J Bone Joint Surg. 2015;97:186–93.
31. Johnson RL, Kopp SL, Burkle CM, Duncan CM, Jacob AK, Erwin PJ, et al. Neuraxial vs general anaesthesia for total hip and total knee arthroplasty: a systematic review of comparative-effectiveness research. Br J Anaesth. 2016;116:163.
32. Turnbull ZA, Sastow D, Giambrone GP, Tedore T. Anesthesia for the patient undergoing total knee replacement: current status and future prospects. Local Reg Anesth. 2017;10:1–7.
33. Weinstein SM, Baaklini LR, Liu J, Poultsides L, Cozowicz C, Poeran J, et al. Neuraxial anaesthesia techniques and postoperative outcomes among joint arthroplasty patients: is spinal anaesthesia the best option? Br J Anaesth. 2018;121(4):842–9.
34. Wyles C, Pagnano MW, Trousdale RT, Sierra RJ, Taunton MJ, Perry KI, et al. Quicker and more predictable return of motor function and ambulation after 1 mepivacaine vs bupivacaine spinal: a double blinded RCT in primary TKAs and THAs. 2019.
35. Pagnano MW, Hebl J, Horlocker T. Assuring a painless total hip arthroplasty: a multimodal approach emphasizing peripheral nerve blocks. J Arthroplast. 2006;21(4 SUPPL):80–4.
36. Ilfeld BM, Duke KB, Donohue MC. The association between lower extremity continuous peripheral nerve blocks and patient falls after knee and hip arthroplasty. Anesth Analg. 2010;111(6):1552–4.
37. Elkassabany NM, Antosh S, Ahmed M, Nelson C, Israelite C, Badiola I, et al. The risk of falls after total knee arthroplasty with the use of a femoral nerve block versus an adductor canal block: a double-blinded randomized controlled study. Anesth Analg. 2016;122(5):1696–703. http://www.ncbi.nlm.nih.gov/pubmed/27007076.
38. Spangehl MJ, Clarke HD, Hentz JG, Misra L, Blocher JL, Seamans DP. The Chitranjan Ranawat award: periarticular injections and femoral & sciatic blocks provide similar pain relief after TKA: a randomized clinical trial. Clin Orthop Relat Res. 2015;473(1):45–53.
39. Elkassabany NM, Cai LF, Badiola I, Kase B, Liu J, Hughes C, et al. A prospective randomized open-label study of single injection versus continuous adductor canal block for postoperative analgesia after total knee arthroplasty. Bone Joint J. 2019;101-B(3):340–7.
40. Amundson AW, Johnson RL, Abdel MP, Mantilla CB, Panchamia JK, Taunton MJ, et al. A three-arm randomized clinical trial comparing continuous femoral plus single-injection sciatic peripheral nerve blocks versus periarticular injection with ropivacaine or liposomal bupivacaine for patients undergoing total knee arthroplasty. Anesthesiology. 2017;126(6):1139–50.

41. Nielsen ND, Runge C, Clemmesen L, Børglum J, Mikkelsen LR, Larsen JR, et al. An obturator nerve block does not alleviate postoperative pain after total hip arthroplasty: a randomized clinical trial. Reg Anesth Pain Med. 2019;44(4):466–71.
42. Johnson RL, Amundson AW, Abdel MP, Sviggum HP, Mabry TM, Mantilla CB, et al. Continuous posterior lumbar plexus nerve block versus periarticular injection with ropivacaine or liposomal bupivacaine for total hip arthroplasty: a three-arm randomized clinical trial. J Bone Joint Surg Am. 2017;99(21):1836–45. http://www.ncbi.nlm.nih.gov/pubmed/29088038.
43. Lombardi AV, Berend KR, Mallory TH, Dodds KL, Adams JB. Soft tissue and intra-articular injection of bupivacaine, epinephrine, and morphine has a beneficial effect after total knee arthroplasty. Clin Orthop Relat Res. 2004;428:125–30. http://www.ncbi.nlm.nih.gov/pubmed/15534532.
44. Talmo CT, Kent SE, Fredette AN, Anderson MC, Hassan MK, Mattingly DA. Prospective randomized trial comparing femoral nerve block with intraoperative local anesthetic injection of liposomal bupivacaine in total knee arthroplasty. J Arthroplast. 2018;33(11):3474–8.
45. Kelley TC, Adams MJ, Mulliken BD, Dalury DF. Efficacy of multimodal perioperative analgesia protocol with periarticular medication injection in total knee arthroplasty: a randomized, double-blinded study. J Arthroplast. 2013;28(8):1274–7.
46. Tsukada S, Kurosaka K, Maeda T, Iida A, Nishino M, Hirasawa N. Early stage periarticular injection during total knee arthroplasty may provide a better postoperative pain relief than late-stage periarticular injection: a randomized-controlled trial. Knee Surg Sports Traumatol Arthrosc. 2019;27(4):1124–31.
47. Jain RK, Porat MD, Klingenstein GG, Reid JJ, Post RE, Schoifet SD. The AAHKS clinical research award: liposomal bupivacaine and periarticular injection are not superior to single-shot intra-articular injection for pain control in Total knee arthroplasty. J Arthroplast. 2016;31(9):22–5.
48. Zlotnicki JP, Hamlin BR, Plakseychuk AY, Levison TJ, Rothenberger SD, Urish KL. Liposomal bupivacaine vs plain bupivacaine in periarticular injection for control of pain and early motion in total knee arthroplasty: a randomized, prospective study. J Arthroplast. 2018;33(8):2460–4.
49. Kuang MJ, Du Y, Ma JX, He W, Fu L, Ma XL. The efficacy of liposomal bupivacaine using periarticular injection in total knee arthroplasty: a systematic review and meta-analysis. J Arthroplast. 2017;32:1395–402.
50. Abdel MP. Mayo Clinic lower extremity multimodal opioid-sparing total joint pathway. 2019.

Chapter 6
Surgical Techniques and Protocols to Minimize Blood Loss and Postoperative Pain

Nathanael Heckmann and Scott Sporer

Introduction

Modern outpatient total joint arthroplasty (TJA) is possible because of recent advances in surgical techniques and perioperative protocols that have decreased blood loss and minimized postoperative pain thereby facilitating more rapid recovery. This has allowed selected patients to go home on the same day of surgery. Historically, TJA was associated with a high rate of blood product transfusion, with national rates ranging from 15–20% following total knee arthroplasty [1] and 24–28% following total hip arthroplasty [2]. Today, with less invasive surgical techniques, hypotensive anesthesia, and the broad utilization of tranexamic acid, transfusion rates have markedly decreased. Furthermore, modern advancements in surgical techniques and postoperative pain protocols have allowed patients to mobilize quicker and return home sooner. Here we describe blood management and surgical techniques surgeons can utilize to safely facilitate outpatient TJA. Multimodal pain protocols and anesthetic techniques including regional blocks are discussed in separate chapters and will not be discussed extensively here.

N. Heckmann
Department of Orthopaedic Surgery, Keck Medical Center of USC, Los Angeles, CA, USA
e-mail: nathanael.heckmann@med.usc.edu

S. Sporer (✉)
Department of Orthopaedic Surgery, Rush University Medical Center, Chicago, IL, USA
e-mail: scott.sporer@rushortho.com

R. M. Meneghini, L. T. Buller (eds.), *Outpatient Hip and Knee Replacement*,
https://doi.org/10.1007/978-3-031-27037-6_6

Blood Management

Preoperative Optimization

Blood management starts with a thorough preoperative evaluation of the patient and involves an assessment of the patient's comorbidities, hemoglobin, and surgical considerations based on the patient's anatomy (i.e., presence of deformity, body habitus, etc.). Prior to surgical intervention, patients should undergo a detailed medical examination that includes a thorough assessment of nutritional status, comorbidity burden, body mass index, as well as other medical factors that may be associated with anemia or increased intraoperative blood loss. Patients with a known or presumptive history of blood dyscrasias, particularly coagulopathies, should be assessed preoperatively by a hematologist for preoperative optimization and perioperative care.

Patients with low starting hemoglobin should be optimized to mitigate their risk of requiring a postoperative blood transfusion. Medical treatment of preoperative anemia should follow a systematic algorithm. First, if a singular underlying cause of the patient's anemia is identified (e.g., iron deficiency), this should be addressed and corrected before elective TJA, if possible. If a patient is determined to have chronic anemia from an irreversible medical condition (e.g., lupus, rheumatoid arthritis, etc.), the surgeon should consider sending the patient to a hematologist or medical specialist for further optimization and management.

In regard to perioperative blood management, several medical strategies exist to optimize a patient preoperatively. Vitamin and mineral supplementation with iron, folate, vitamin C, and vitamin B_{12} may help correct certain types of anemias, particularly if the anemia is caused by a specific vitamin or mineral deficiency. Vitamin supplementation preoperatively may also provide the patient with ideal "building blocks" to undergo postoperative hematopoiesis in a potentially more efficient way. However, there is limited data about the clinical benefit of vitamin supplementation in patients with normal preoperative hemoglobin [3–5]. A study by Cuenca et al. assessed 156 consecutive patients who received ferrous sulfate (256 mg/day), vitamin C (1000 mg/day), and folic acid (5 mg/day) for 30–45 days before undergoing a primary total knee replacement [3]. The authors of this study noted a decrease in transfusion rates in patients who received vitamin supplementation from 32% to 5.8%. However, the authors did not use tranexamic acid, used tourniquets that were let down after skin closure, and used two deep drains in all patients, limiting the generalizability of their findings. Currently, there are no high-quality data supporting the routine preoperative supplementation of all patients with vitamins and minerals. As such, preoperative supplementation should be done on a case-by-case basis, particularly for patients with preoperative anemia and a known deficiency.

Erythropoietin supplementation may also be utilized for patients with preoperative anemia prior to surgery. While routine use of preoperative erythropoietin supplementation is not supported by the literature, its use for select cases where large amounts of anticipated blood loss are expected and for patients with preoperative anemia may be warranted. A study by Pierson et al. used erythropoietin in select patients as part of a blood-conservation strategy in 500 consecutive patients undergoing primary total knee or total hip arthroplasty and reported a transfusion rate of 2.1% compared to 16.4% in a group that did not follow the author's algorithm [6]. However, the authors of this study did not use tranexamic acid, limiting the applicability of their findings to current clinical practice. Other authors have reported decreased blood loss and lower transfusion rates associated with the preoperative administration of erythropoietin in select patients [7, 8].

Lastly, preoperative autologous donation of blood products may be considered in patients with preoperative anemia or if more than typical blood loss is expected at the time of surgery. While this strategy was used frequently in the past with variable efficacy, preoperative screening and optimization as well as the near-universal use of tranexamic acid have led to a marked decrease in this practice [9]. As such, preoperative autologous donation of blood products should be used only for select cases, particularly when large amounts of blood loss are expected, scenarios that are almost always reserved for the inpatient surgical setting and thus not applicable to outpatient surgery.

Intraoperative Blood Management Strategies

Intraoperative blood management strategies include tourniquet use during total knee arthroplasty (TKA), electrocautery, less invasive surgical techniques, antifibrinolytic medication, and hemostatic agents. While the merits of tourniquet use during primary TKA is currently a subject of debate, several studies have documented improved visualization, increased operative efficiency, decreased operative time, improved cement interdigitation, decreased blood loss, and decreased rates of postoperative transfusion [10, 11]. However, some surgeons advocate against the use of tourniquets during routine primary TKA, citing increased pain and swelling, decreased quadriceps strength, and cellular damage related to transient ischemia. In today's climate of broad tranexamic use, the prior debates about the merits of tourniquet use as a means to decrease blood loss may be diminished and it remains the surgeon's choice based upon the level of surgical comfort.

The broad utilization of tranexamic acid had led to less blood loss and markedly decreased rates of allogeneic blood transfusion following primary total hip and total knee arthroplasty. In the past, high rates of transfusion in TJA mandated inpatient observation. Recent guidelines from the American Academy of Hip and Knee Surgeons, American Society of Regional Anesthesia and Pain Medicine, American Academy of Orthopaedic Surgeons, The Hip Society, and The Knee Society now recommend tranexamic acid administration for knee and hip arthroplasty as a means of decreasing blood loss and reducing the risk of transfusion [12]. These guidelines do not recommend a specific route of administration, citing insufficient data to recommend between intravenous, oral, topical, or a combination thereof. Rather, the guidelines recommend that a dose of tranexamic acid be given, regardless of route, prior to skin incision as an effective means to decrease blood transfusion rates. Lastly, the guidelines cite a lack of sufficient data to support multiple doses of tranexamic acid utilization. If there is one takeaway from this chapter, it is that all patients should receive tranexamic acid in the perioperative period unless there is a true contraindication to its administration.

Postoperative Pain

Tourniquet Use

In the discussion of postoperative surgical pain, one of the more commonly debated topics is tourniquet use. As mentioned previously, tourniquet use during TKA remains popular among surgeons due to improved visualization, reduced intraoperative blood loss, and improved cement mantle. However, the resultant ischemia has been associated with increased postoperative pain [13–16]. As such, some surgeons advocate for tourniquet-less surgery, in which it is only used during cementation, as a means to decrease postoperative pain and promote more rapid functional recovery. However, the evidence is conflicting as some studies failed to detect a difference in postoperative pain levels among patients undergoing TKA with or without tourniquet use [11, 17, 18]. A double-blinded randomized study by Goel et al. assessed 200 patients undergoing elective TKA and randomized them to undergo surgery with or without a tourniquet [11]. The authors of this study reported greater blood loss and decreased surgical visualization in the group that did not receive a tourniquet, and did find any difference between the two groups in regard to pain, range of motion, or function.

While the topic of tourniquet use merits further investigation, some limited evidence points to the notion that it may not necessarily be the use of tourniquets but rather the manner in which they are used. One such possible concept is to use the tourniquet for a shorter period of time, which was shown in a randomized trial to reduce postoperative pain [19]. Considering most surgeons' operative speed is not easily modified, if shorter tourniquet time is desired, it is best to target its use to maximize the benefit. Most techniques utilizing short tourniquet time focus on the cementation portion to maximize the cement mantle and therefore the durability of the reconstruction [16]. A recent meta-analysis of randomized controlled trials found that cement-only tourniquet application resulted in greater blood loss, but improved postoperative pain and earlier functional recovery [20]. The study was limited by the general lack of high-quality trials investigating pain specifically. More research is required on this topic, particularly in light of the increasing popularity of uncemented TKAs, where improving the cement mantle is not a consideration.

Tranexamic Acid

The utilization of tranexamic acid has rapidly increased in popularity in TJA as a means to reduce blood loss and minimize the need for subsequent transfusion. However, another benefit of this medication may be the ability to reduce early postoperative pain by decreasing the size and duration of postoperative hemarthrosis. By reducing the volume and duration of postoperative hemarthrosis, patients may experience less pressure within the joint, allowing for decreased pain and improved early range of motion. While the association between tranexamic acid use and decreased pain is a relatively new concept that has been demonstrated in other orthopedic specialties, particularly in anterior cruciate ligament reconstruction surgery, this relationship has not been demonstrated in TJA.

Several well-powered randomized controlled trials have shown that tranexamic acid given during anterior cruciate ligament reconstruction surgery significantly reduces postoperative hemarthrosis and pain, along with the expected reduction in blood loss [21–23]. However, limited data exists supporting a relationship between tranexamic use and decreased postoperative pain in arthroplasty patients. Wang et al. conducted a double-blinded prospective randomized controlled trial in patients undergoing primary TKA [24]. All patients received pre-incision and 3-h postsurgical intravenous tranexamic acid,and were then randomized to receive oral tranexamic acid or placebo for 14 days. The authors noted decreased ecchymosis and swelling in the group that received prolonged oral tranexamic acid, but were unable to demonstrate any differences in pain. However, the study was not powered to detect differences in pain scores. A recent retrospective study by Grosso et al. found improved pain levels during physical therapy in patients who received tranexamic acid during TKA [25]. The authors of this study found that patients who received tranexamic acid were able to ambulate approximately 20% more than patients who did not receive this intervention. However, the retrospective nature of this study is subject to confounding and bias, highlighting the need for further high-powered studies before any definitive conclusion can be made between pain relief and tranexamic acid utilization.

Incision Length and Surgical Technique

Surgical technique may play a crucial role in postoperative pain and recovery. One technical aspect that was previously thought to influence pain is the length of the skin incision, as more pain fibers are likely recruited by increasing incisional length, suggesting smaller "minimally invasive" incisions may result in improved pain and postoperative outcome. However, there is currently limited data to support this notion [26]. A recent retrospective study by Nam et al. analyzed over 1800 patients who underwent elective total hip arthroplasty and were unable to demonstrate a relationship between incision length and postoperative pain [27]. A meta-analysis by Xu et al. encompassing 14 studies and over 1100 THA patients found no difference in pain medication dosing postoperatively based on incision length [28].

While incision length alone may not provide any marked differences in postoperative pain, other aspects of so-called minimally invasive TJA may lead to decreased postoperative pain and improved early functional recovery, such as decreased deep dissection and less traumatic exposure technique. A study by Dorr et al. randomized patients undergoing elective total hip arthroplasty to a minimally invasive 10 cm incision group or a traditional long incision 20 cm group. At the end of the case, the surgeon extended the incision length of the minimally invasive group to match the incision length of the long incision group. The patients in the minimally invasive group had improved early postoperative pain and shorter inpatient length of stay. The authors of this study noted that the minimally invasive group underwent less extensive splitting of the gluteus maximus and less extensive deep dissection, suggesting that the benefits conferred by minimally invasive surgery may be related to the extent of the deeper soft tissue manipulation rather than the length of the skin incision. Another study by Majima et al. assessed 200 consecutive elective TKA patients who were randomized to a minimally invasive patellar subluxation group or a traditional extensile patellar eversion group [29]. The authors found that the minimally invasive group had decreased postoperative pain and better postoperative motion and improved postoperative strength. These studies suggest that factors other than skin incision length have an effect on postoperative pain and recovery.

However, the data regarding minimally invasive surgery and postoperative pain is mixed, largely due to limitations in the ability to accurately measure and standardize the extent of deeper soft tissue dissection, limitations in the sensitivity of instruments available to measure pain, and the subjective nature of pain perception by surgical patients. One small randomized trial found no difference in early postoperative Knee Society Scores and Western Ontario and McMaster Universities Osteoarthritis Index (WOMAC) scores between conventional and minimally invasive TKA patients [30]. In contrast, a single-surgeon study found a minimally invasive technique was associated with both improved range of motion and decreased pain scores compared to a standard incision in patients undergoing elective total knee arthroplasty [31]. This was corroborated in a smaller study, which found that smaller incisions were associated with improved pain scores and decreased pain medication usage, but were also associated with a higher incidence of varus malalignment of the tibial component possibly due to reduced visualization [32]. More research is needed to assess what aspects of minimally invasive surgery lead to less pain without compromising component position or implant longevity.

The surgical technique during TKA exposure may affect postoperative pain. A small study comparing a minimally invasive midvastus approach to a standard medial parapatellar incision found that the midvastus approach was associated with reduced pain scores and decreased pain medication use [33]. This was confirmed in a small randomized study, which found a similar, mini-subvastus approach resulted in reduced pain and improved functional outcome scores compared to the standard approach [34]. In contrast, a randomized double-blinded trial in patients undergoing TKA found no difference in postoperative pain between a midvastus and standard medial parapatellar approach [35]. However, this trial was performed in simultaneous bilateral TKA patients, with a different approach performed on each side limiting the generalizability of these findings.

Conclusion

Advances in blood management and surgical technique for TJA have led to decreased blood loss, lower rates of transfusion, decreased pain, and accelerated postoperative recovery, facilitating same-day discharge. Further study is needed to elucidate the technical aspects of minimally invasive surgery that lead to the most benefit in terms of decreasing postoperative pain. Within the context of outpatient TJA, surgeons should utilize tranexamic acid on all patients and choose a surgical technique they are most comfortable with to reduce surgical times and hasten their patient's recovery.

References

1. Klika AK, Small TJ, Saleh A, Szubski CR, Chandran Pillai ALP, Barsoum WK. Primary total knee arthroplasty allogenic transfusion trends, length of stay, and complications: nationwide inpatient sample 2000-2009. J Arthroplast. 2014;29(11):2070–7.
2. Saleh A, Small T, Chandran Pillai ALP, Schiltz NK, Klika AK, Barsoum WK. Allogenic blood transfusion following total hip arthroplasty: results from the nationwide inpatient sample, 2000 to 2009. J Bone Joint Surg Am. 2014;96(18):e155.
3. Cuenca J, García-Erce JA, Martínez F, Cardona R, Pérez-Serrano L, Muñoz M. Preoperative haematinics and transfusion protocol reduce the need for transfusion after total knee replacement. Int J Surg. 2007;5(2):89–94.
4. García-Erce JA, Cuenca J, Martínez F, Cardona R, Pérez-Serrano L, Muñoz M. Perioperative intravenous iron preserves iron stores and may hasten the recovery from post-operative anaemia after knee replacement surgery. Transfus Med. 2006;16(5):335–41.
5. Cuenca J, García-Erce JA, Martínez F, Pérez-Serrano L, Herrera A, Muñoz M. Perioperative intravenous iron, with or without erythropoietin, plus restrictive transfusion protocol reduce the need for allogeneic blood after knee replacement surgery. Transfusion. 2006;46(7):1112–9.
6. Pierson JL, Hannon TJ, Earles DR. A blood-conservation algorithm to reduce blood transfusions after total hip and knee arthroplasty. J Bone Joint Surg Am. 2004;86(7):1512–8.
7. Bezwada HP, Nazarian DG, Henry DH, Booth RE Jr. Preoperative use of recombinant human erythropoietin before total joint arthroplasty. J Bone Joint Surg Am. 2003;85(9):1795–800.
8. Deutsch A, Spaulding J, Marcus RE. Preoperative epoetin alfa vs autologous blood donation in primary total knee arthroplasty. J Arthroplast. 2006;21(5):628–35.
9. Abdel MP, Berry DJ. Current practice trends in primary hip and knee arthroplasties among members of the American Association of hip and Knee Surgeons: a long-term update. J Arthroplast. 2019;34(7):S24–7. https://doi.org/10.1016/j.arth.2019.02.006.
10. Tai T-W, Chang C-W, Lai K-A, Lin C-J, Yang C-Y. Effects of tourniquet use on blood loss and soft-tissue damage in total knee arthroplasty: a randomized controlled trial. J Bone Joint Surg Am. 2012;94(24):2209–15.

11. Goel R, Rondon AJ, Sydnor K, et al. Tourniquet use does not affect functional outcomes or pain after total knee arthroplasty: a prospective, double-blinded, randomized controlled trial. J Bone Joint Surg Am. 2019;101(20):1821–8.
12. Fillingham YA, Ramkumar DB, Jevsevar DS, et al. Tranexamic acid use in total joint arthroplasty: the clinical practice guidelines endorsed by the American Association of hip and knee surgeons, American Society of regional anesthesia and pain medicine, American Academy of orthopaedic surgeons, hip society, and knee society. J Arthroplast. 2018;33(10):3065–9.
13. Kheir MM, Ziemba-Davis M, Dilley JE, Hood MJ, Meneghini RM. Tourniquetless Total knee arthroplasty with modern perioperative protocols decreases pain and opioid consumption in women. J Arthroplast. 2018;33(11):3455–9.
14. Zhou K, Ling T, Wang H, et al. Influence of tourniquet use in primary total knee arthroplasty with drainage: a prospective randomised controlled trial. J Orthop Surg Res. 2017;12(1):172.
15. Liu Y, Si H, Zeng Y, Li M, Xie H, Shen B. More pain and slower functional recovery when a tourniquet is used during total knee arthroplasty. Knee Surg Sports Traumatol Arthrosc. 2020;28(6):1842–60.
16. Pfitzner T, von Roth P, Voerkelius N, Mayr H, Perka C, Hube R. Influence of the tourniquet on tibial cement mantle thickness in primary total knee arthroplasty. Knee Surg Sports Traumatol Arthrosc. 2016;24(1):96–101.
17. Dong J, Min S, He K-H, Peng L-H, Cao J, Ran W. Effects of the nontourniquet combined with controlled hypotension technique on pain and long-term prognosis in elderly patients after total knee arthroplasty: a randomized controlled study. J Anesth. 2019;33(5):587–93.
18. Barker T, Rogers VE, Brown KB, Henriksen VT, Rasmussen GL. Tourniquet use during total knee arthroplasty does not modulate the neutrophil-to-lymphocyte ratio, pain, or activity. J Orthop Traumatol. 2017;18(3):283–7.
19. Wang K, Ni S, Li Z, et al. The effects of tourniquet use in total knee arthroplasty: a randomized, controlled trial. Knee Surg Sports Traumatol Arthrosc. 2017;25(9):2849–57.
20. Wang C, Zhou C, Qu H, Yan S, Pan Z. Comparison of tourniquet application only during cementation and long-duration tourniquet application in total knee arthroplasty: a meta-analysis. J Orthop Surg Res. 2018;13(1):216.
21. Karaaslan F, Karaoğlu S, Yurdakul E. Reducing intra-articular Hemarthrosis after arthroscopic anterior cruciate ligament reconstruction by the administration of intravenous tranexamic acid: a prospective, randomized controlled trial. Am J Sports Med. 2015;43(11):2720–6.
22. Chiang E-R, Chen K-H, Wang S-T, et al. Intra-articular injection of tranexamic acid reduced postoperative hemarthrosis in arthroscopic anterior cruciate ligament reconstruction: a prospective randomized study. Arthroscopy. 2019;35(7):2127–32.
23. Felli L, Revello S, Burastero G, et al. Single intravenous administration of tranexamic acid in anterior cruciate ligament reconstruction to reduce postoperative hemarthrosis and increase functional outcomes in the early phase of postoperative rehabilitation: a randomized controlled trial. Arthroscopy. 2019;35(1):149–57.
24. Wang H-Y, Wang L, Luo Z-Y, et al. Intravenous and subsequent long-term oral tranexamic acid in enhanced-recovery primary total knee arthroplasty without the application of a tourniquet: a randomized placebo-controlled trial. BMC Musculoskelet Disord. 2019;20(1):478.
25. Grosso MJ, Trofa DP, Danoff JR, et al. Tranexamic acid increases early perioperative functional outcomes after total knee arthroplasty. Arthroplast Today. 2018;4(1):74–7.
26. Lloyd JM, Wainwright T, Middleton RG. What is the role of minimally invasive surgery in a fast track hip and knee replacement pathway? Ann R Coll Surg Engl. 2012;94(3):148–51.
27. Nam D, Nunley RM, Clohisy JC, Lombardi AV, Berend KR, Barrack RL. Does patient-reported perception of pain differ based on surgical approach in total hip arthroplasty? Bone Joint J. 2019;101-B(6_Supple_B):31–6.
28. Xu C-P, Li X, Song J-Q, Cui Z, Yu B. Mini-incision versus standard incision total hip arthroplasty regarding surgical outcomes: a systematic review and meta-analysis of randomized controlled trials. PLoS One. 2013;8(11):e80021.

29. Majima T, Nishiike O, Sawaguchi N, Susuda K, Minami A. Patella eversion reduces early knee range of motion and muscle torque recovery after total knee arthroplasty: comparison between minimally invasive total knee arthroplasty and conventional total knee arthroplasty. Arthritis. 2011;2011:854651.
30. Lüring C, Beckmann J, Haiböck P, Perlick L, Grifka J, Tingart M. Minimal invasive and computer assisted total knee replacement compared with the conventional technique: a prospective, randomised trial. Knee Surg Sports Traumatol Arthrosc. 2008;16(10):928–34.
31. McAllister CM, Stepanian JD. The impact of minimally invasive surgical techniques on early range of motion after primary total knee arthroplasty. J Arthroplast. 2008;23(1):10–8.
32. Dalury DF, Dennis DA. Mini-incision total knee arthroplasty can increase risk of component malalignment. Clin Orthop Relat Res. 2005;440:77–81.
33. Laskin RS, Beksac B, Phongjunakorn A, et al. Minimally invasive total knee replacement through a mini-midvastus incision: an outcome study. Clin Orthop Relat Res. 2004;428:74–81.
34. Li Z, Cheng W, Sun L, et al. Mini-subvastus versus medial parapatellar approach for total knee arthroplasty: a prospective randomized controlled study. Int Orthop. 2018;42(3):543–9.
35. Nestor BJ, Toulson CE, Backus SI, Lyman SL, Foote KL, Windsor RE. Mini-midvastus vs standard medial parapatellar approach: a prospective, randomized, double-blinded study in patients undergoing bilateral total knee arthroplasty. J Arthroplast. 2010;25(6 Suppl):5–11. 11.e1

Chapter 7
Anesthesia for Outpatient TJA: Anesthetic Techniques and Regional Blocks

Mark E. Nielson

Preoperatively

Patient Optimization

Following safe patient selection for outpatient TJA [1, 2], preoperative optimization of patient physical status and comorbidities helps to insure a successful outpatient surgery. At our institution, we achieve this goal by using a single internal medicine physician who works only with TJA patients to prepare them for surgery and medically follow them after surgery. In addition, upcoming surgeries are discussed during a routine coordinated care conference attended by all key members of the multidisciplinary care team. The goal of the meeting is to share information across disciplines, anticipate and answer questions, and proactively develop patient care plans based on comorbidities and needs.

Institutions also have adopted Enhanced Recovery After Surgery (ERAS) protocols to maximize optimal recovery following major surgery [3]. Important aspects of ERAS protocols are preoperative nutrition, preoperative fluid status, multimodal pain protocols, and early mobilization. The main objectives for fluid status and nutrition remain the same for the reduction of postoperative insulin resistance [3]. Nutritional status should be addressed with increased protein intake if appropriate, and fluid carbohydrate loading is appropriate for up to 2 h prior to surgery. This helps to optimize fluid status and reduces the immediate risk from a catabolic state.

M. E. Nielson (✉)
Indiana University Health Saxony Hospital, Fishers, IN, USA
e-mail: mnielson@aci-llc.net

R. M. Meneghini, L. T. Buller (eds.), *Outpatient Hip and Knee Replacement*,
https://doi.org/10.1007/978-3-031-27037-6_7

Multimodal Pain Control

The nervous system is an intricate system of pain, pressure, and proprioceptive sensors connected to signal transducing tissue. Signals are transmitted from the peripheral tissues to the brain via a pain pathway. Medications can act along many areas of the signaling pathway. Multimodal analgesia permits a reduction of opioids and therefore opioid-related side effects by targeting different pain receptors along the pathway with different medications. Large doses of any one drug, especially those with sedative effects, should be avoided in the outpatient setting. Some of the most common medications used in multimodal pathways are summarized below along with their mechanisms and sites of action.

Analgesics: Acetaminophen is an analgesic. Its exact mechanism of action is not known. It is theorized however to inhibit prostaglandin synthesis as well as the activation of descending serotonergic pathways in the brain. Its effect is mainly central.

Nonsteroidal Anti-Inflammatory Drugs (NSAIDs): NSAIDs work by inhibiting the activity of cyclooxygenase enzymes. This in turn inhibits the synthesis of prostaglandins and thromboxanes from arachidonic acid. Their anti-inflammatory effect is seen in the peripheral tissues but they also have central effects on the descending pain control system.

Opioids: Opioids produce their pharmacologic actions by acting on receptors located on neuronal cell membranes. Pain relief is thought to be due to the mu receptor. They inhibit presynaptic neurotransmitter release. The site of action is both central and peripheral (Fig. 7.1).

Gabanoids: Pregabalin and Gabapentin are the main gabanoids used in multimodal pain regimens. They exert their effects by inhibiting the alpha 2 delta subunit of voltage-gated calcium channels. They have anti-hyperalgesic and anti-allodynic effects. The site of action is both peripheral and central.

Antiemetics: Nausea and vomiting are mediated primarily by visceral stimulation through dopamine and serotonin. The neurotransmitters histamine (H), acetylcholine, serotonin, and dopamine frequently are implicated in nausea and vomiting and are the targets of most therapeutic modalities [5].

- Famotidine blocks H2 receptors. It has no direct antiemetic effect but reduces acid secretion by up to 90%.
- Ondansetron is a serotonin antagonist with central activity.
- Promethazine is a weak dopamine receptor antagonist and H1 receptor blocker. It has both central and peripheral effects.
- Dexamethasone's antiemetic mechanism is not understood but it is theorized to have direct central action at the solitary tract nucleus, interaction with the neurotransmitter serotonin, and the receptor proteins tachykinin NK1 and NK2, alpha-adrenaline. It has both central and peripheral effects. Of note, the antiemetic effect of dexamethasone is greater if given at the start, rather than the end, of surgery. It has a half-life of over 50 h and thus some institutions avoid its use because patients are in a state of postsurgical insulin resistance after surgery. Some studies show an increased risk while others do not [6, 7].

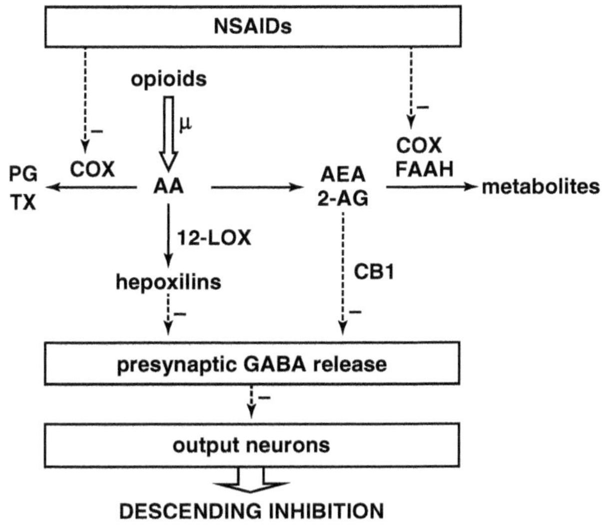

Fig. 7.1 "Proposed model for the interaction of NSAIDs, opioids, and cannabinoids in the descending pain control system to induce analgesia. Minus symbols indicate inhibition. Inhibition of the cyclooxygenases (COX) by NSAIDs reduces the synthesis of prostaglandins (PG) and thromboxanes (TX) and thus increases the availability of arachidonic acid (AA). Opioids also increase the availability of AA by activating the phospholipase A_2 via the μ-opioid receptor. Via the 12-lipoxygenases (12-LOX) AA is transformed into hepoxilins, which indirectly inhibit GABA release. By inhibiting COX and FAAH the NSAIDs spare AEA and 2-AG, which bind to the CB1 receptor (The role of the CB2 receptor in this model has not been established.) and thus inhibit GABA release. Removal of inhibition by GABA enhances the activity of output neurons that inhibit pain" [4]. (Source: https://www.mdpi.com/1424-8247/3/5/1335. License: Creative Commons Attribution License https://creativecommons.org/licenses/by-nc-sa/3.0/legalcode)

- Prochlorperazine's mechanism of action is unknown but it is believed to block dopamine in the brain.
- Essential oils: There are proprietary blends of essential oils that when inhaled have been shown to have antiemetic effects. The exact mechanism of action is unknown.
- Scopolamine is an anticholinergic. It acts as a competitive inhibitor at postganglionic muscarinic receptor sites of the parasympathetic nervous system. It also acts on smooth muscles that respond to acetylcholine but lack cholinergic innervation.
- Anti-Anxiety: Benzodiazepines bind the alpha and gamma subunits of the gaba-a receptor. This increases chloride ion channel opening and increases inhibitory effects of gaba on neuronal excitability. Effects are mainly central. Midazolam has been shown in one study to improve post-op nausea [8].

Intraoperatively

Evidence-based guidelines for the best primary anesthetic have yet to be elucidated. Several studies have shown that spinal anesthesia has fewer complications and side effects than general anesthesia. However, current clinical trials are questioning these results. The decision to use spinal anesthesia, general anesthesia, or a combination of both should be made on a program-by-program basis. The needs of each program are influenced by both surgeon and anesthesia experience and preference [9].

Spinal Anesthesia

Several studies have shown benefits from a spinal anesthetic. Decreased blood loss, decreased nausea and vomiting, decreased length of stay, decreased incidence of deep vein thrombosis, increased tissue oxygenation, and thus possible decreased infection rates have all been demonstrated [10]. According to 2014 American College of Cardiology/American Heart Association guidelines on cardiovascular evaluation and management of patients undergoing non-cardiac surgery, there is no difference in the incidence of myocardial infarction or death when spinal or general anesthesia is used [11]. There are nonetheless multiple factors to consider if a spinal anesthetic is chosen.

Timing: Metabolism and redistribution of anesthetics begin when a spinal is placed limiting the amount of time a patient is rendered insensate from the local anesthetic. If the duration is a concern, a combined spinal and epidural may be performed. Hyperbaric bupivacaine 0.75% is the local anesthetic of choice for most anesthesiologists for spinal anesthesia. However, more recently, different local anesthetics have been chosen for their pharmacokinetic and pharmacodynamic profiles as briefly summarized below. The approximate duration of action based on the dosage of each anesthetic is provided in Table 7.1.

Table 7.1 Approximate duration of local anesthetics based on dose

Local anesthetic	Dose in milligrams	Approximate duration in minutes
Bupivacaine	6	45–75
	7.5	75–90
	10	100–150
	12	150–180
Mepivacaine	39	50–60
	42	60–70
	45	80–90
	50	100–120
Lidocaine	50	100–120
Chloroprocaine	50	60

- Bupivacaine in an intermediate duration amide local anesthetic. It is most commonly seen in a hyperbaric formulation of 0.75% but some institutions use the isobaric 0.5% formulation. It is the most commonly used spinal anesthetic partially due to its low incidence of transient neurologic symptoms.
- Mepivacaine is a short duration amide local anesthetic. It is found in the isobaric form both in 2% and 1.5% formulations. It is noteworthy that intrathecal use of mepivacaine is off label. There has been a recent resurgence of its use as an intrathecal anesthetic with a low incidence of transient neurologic symptoms.
- Lidocaine is a short acting amide local anesthetic. Preservative-free lidocaine can be readily found in 1% and 2% formulations. Some anesthesiologists avoid lidocaine due to its history of a higher incidence of transient neurologic symptoms than bupivacaine and mepivacaine. However, it has been used recently as a short acting local anesthetic with a low reported incidence of transient neurologic symptoms [12].
- Chloroprocaine has FDA clearance as an ultra-short-acting local anesthetic for intrathecal use. It is found in a 1% formulation and is an ester. The incidence of transient neurologic symptoms with chloroprocaine is low.

Opioids in Spinal Anesthesia: The addition of an opioid to intrathecal local anesthetic can have a synergistic effect on analgesia duration. Hydrophilic opioids like morphine have a biphasic effect on respiratory depression that can last up to 24 h. Consequently, morphine is not indicated for outpatient procedures. Lipophilic opioids like fentanyl do not have the same respiratory profile. Fentanyl, which also extends the duration of local spinal anesthesia, has been shown to be safe. Some studies report an increased incidence of urinary retention with the addition of any opioid to the spinal anesthetic. However, fentanyl has been used extensively in the outpatient setting for many years without significant consequences [13, 14]. The typical dose of fentanyl is 15–25 μg in the local solution which may add an additional 15–30 min of time to local anesthesia duration.

Transient Neurologic Symptoms: The prevalence of transient neurologic symptoms (TNS) has driven the decision to use one local anesthetic over another. Lidocaine has the highest listed incidence of TNS and bupivacaine the lowest. The relevance of this in TJA is unclear.

Spinal Headache: A low cerebral spinal fluid (CSF) headache may develop after spinal anesthesia. The mechanism is leaking CSF following a dural puncture. The resulting decrease in CSF causes a gravity-related drag on the brain when standing or sitting which improves while lying flat. The incidence of spinal headache is lower in older patients and higher in younger patients. Consequently, CSF headache is relatively rare in TJA because most patients are older. The incidence of spinal headache is also influenced by the type of needle used. Incidence is higher with a cutting needle and lower with a pencil point needle. It is recommended a pencil point needle be used.

Coagulation Status: Spinal anesthesia is contraindicated if a patient is in an anticoagulated state. The American Society of Regional Anesthesia (ASRA) has provided guidelines for anesthesia in these patients [15]. If a patient is not at an acceptable risk per ASEA guidelines, spinal anesthesia should not be performed.

General Anesthesia

A common misconception is that general anesthesia is only performed with inhalational anesthetics. General anesthesia is a level of sedation and is not defined solely by the type of drug used. The American Society of Anesthesiologists defines general anesthesia as a drug-induced loss of consciousness where patients are not arousable to painful stimulation and often require assistance in maintaining an airway and positive pressure ventilation may be required [16].

Pros of General Anesthesia: General anesthesia can be continuously given to a patient and thus timing/duration of the anesthetic is not an issue. There also are no contraindications related to coagulation status. The failure rate for administering general anesthesia is virtually zero as a secured airway, either by a supraglottic airway or endotracheal tube, is all that is needed. General anesthesia can be administered without a secure airway but is not recommended because the risk of aspiration is increased. General anesthesia poses little to no concern regarding the patient's level of sedation and awareness during surgery, and patients quickly return to normal neurologic function.

Cons of General Anesthesia: General anesthetic blunts the response to surgical stimuli, but it does not render a patient completely insensate. Physical responses to surgery-related changes in heart rate and blood pressure can occur with the latter contributing to blood loss. Treatment of iatrogenic hypertension in the post-anesthetic care unit can present additional challenges and lingering antihypertensive medications may result in hypotension. In addition, an unconscious patient may move in response to surgical stimuli. Paralytics can be used, but they hinder the immediate detection of nervous tissue damage. There is a greater incidence of nausea and vomiting with general anesthesia, in particular general anesthesia utilizing inhalational anesthetics.

Regional Anesthesia for the Hip

Regional anesthesia blocks peripheral nerves in a specific region of the body such as the hip joint. The anteromedial joint capsule of the hip is innervated by the obturator nerve; the anterior joint capsule is innervated by the femoral nerve; and the posteromedial capsule is innervated by the sciatic nerve and articular branches from the sciatic nerve to the quadratus femoris muscle. Articular branches of the superior gluteal nerve innervate the posterolateral joint capsule. The skin and superficial tissues for surgical access are innervated by the lateral femoral cutaneous nerve [17]. Five common regional anesthesia nerve blocks for the hip are described below.

- Facia iliaca compartment blocks have shown good pain control after hip surgery in multiple studies [18]. This block represents an anterior approach to lumbar plexus blocks. A suprainguinal approach placing 30–40 mL of local anesthetic just below the iliacus fascia reliably anesthetizes the femoral, lateral femoral cutaneous, and obturator nerves. Some anesthesiologists have tried using low concentrations of ropivacaine to avoid quadriceps weakness with variable results. Whenever the femoral nerve is anesthetized, muscle weakness can be an issue.
- Quadratus lumborum blocks have been shown to provide pain control after total hip arthroplasty while maintaining adequate muscle strength [19]. This block is similar to the transversus abdominis plane block except local anesthetic is placed posterolateral to the transversus abdominis muscle and just below the fascia of the quadratus lumborum. Clinical trials are underway to help determine the usefulness of this block in the outpatient setting.
- Erector spinae blocks also have been shown to provide pain control after total hip arthroplasty, with adequate strength maintained. Local anesthetic is placed below the erector spinae muscles at the Lumbar 4 transverse process on the ipsilateral side of the surgery. One study showed benefit in pain control as compared to a standard intravenous pain medication regimen [20]. Further studies are needed to determine the utility of this block.
- Lateral femoral cutaneous blocks have been shown to be effective for patients with moderate to severe pain following total hip arthroplasty. It is primarily used as a rescue block. The block is performed by ultrasound landmarks of the tensor fascia lata and the sartorious muscle. The nerve can be visualized close to these structures below the lateral edge of the inguinal ligament.
- Local infiltrative anesthesia (LIA) has been shown to improve pain scores when compared to placebo. However, for hip replacement surgery, LIA is not better than preoperative spinal anesthesia followed by multimodal analgesia with acetaminophen plus an NSAID/COX-2 inhibitor and either glucocorticoid or gabapentinoid [21].

Regional Anesthesia for the Knee

Peripheral nerve blocks are commonly used in total knee arthroplasty. The anterior knee capsule is innervated by the prepatellar plexus which consists of quadrants. The superolateral quadrant is innervated by the nerve to the vastus lateralis, the nerve to the vastus intermedius, superior lateral genicular nerves, and common fibular nerves. The inferolateral quadrant is innervated by inferior lateral genicular nerves and recurrent fibular nerves. The superomedial quadrant is innervated by nerves to the vastus lateralis, vastus medialis, vastus intermedius, and the superior medial genicular nerves. The inferomedial quadrant is innervated by inferior medial genicular nerves and the infrapatellar branch of the saphenous nerve [22]. The posterior knee capsule is innervated by the obturator, tibial, and common fibular nerves.

Regional blocks commonly used for anterior knee pain include:

- Femoral nerve blocks were traditionally the gold standard for pain control after total knee arthroplasty. A high incidence of quadriceps weakness creating fall risks and delayed rehabilitation after surgery have resulted in decreased use of this block in the inpatient setting and virtually nonexistent use in the outpatient setting.
- Adductor canal block has become the new gold standard in knee arthroplasty because it provides equivalent pain control as femoral nerve block and is less likely to reduce strength in the quadriceps muscle. The block is performed by placing local anesthetic in the adductor canal below the sartorious muscle at the mid to distal thigh. The vastoadductor fascia must be pierced by the needle or local anesthetic may not reach the canal appropriately. The saphenous nerve, nerve to the vastus medialis, and branches of the obturator nerve are reliably in the canal. Proximal spread of local anesthetic may be seen in up to 58% of patients. Whether the spread is clinically significant differs with each patient. At our institution, clinically significant quadriceps weakness was observed in 9% (92/1021) of patients (unpublished data). 20 mL appears to be the appropriate dose to fill the canal [23]. Pointing the ultrasound transducer as well as the needle obliquely distal during injection theoretically places the local in a more distal location.

  Single shot adductor canal blocks require less equipment and follow-up and do not require removal of equipment or post-procedural management. Continuous adductor canal blocks may provide additional pain control 24–48 h after surgery but recent studies are contradictory [24]. A recently published randomized control trial showed single shot and continuous adductor canal blocks to be virtually equivocal [25].

- Local Infiltrative Anesthesia includes periarticular injection which has been shown to provide good pain control following knee arthroplasty when compared to placebo [26]. Timing of the periarticular injection prior to arthrotomy rather than following component implantation may also play a role in optimizing pain control [27]. A recent study showed that periarticular injection provided better pain relief than adductor canal block alone [28]. It is important to note however that pain scores did not differ in the two groups on postoperative day 0. Postoperative day 1 showed the difference. Local adjuncts to extend the duration of analgesia were not used so neither the adductor canal block nor the periarticular injection would be expected to last more than 8–12 h given that the half-life of bupivacaine is 2.7 h. Another study showed that the addition of an adductor canal block improved pain and opioid consumption beyond that provided by periarticular injection [29]. There are many different formulations with adjuncts for periarticular injection. An example of a common formulation is Ropivacaine 200 mg, Ketorolac 30 mg, Clonidine 80 μg, and Epinephrine 0.5 mg in a total of 101.3 mL solution.

Regional blocks commonly used for posterior knee pain include:

- iPACK (Infiltration between Popliteal Artery and Capsule of the Knee) blocks have emerged as effective means of providing pain control without significant side effects. Local anesthetic is placed under ultrasound guidance between the capsule of the knee and the popliteal artery. Articular branches of the tibial nerve are anesthetized. Foot drop due to sciatic spread of local anesthetic can occur but reported incidence is low.
- Spank (Sensory Posterior Articular Nerves of the Knee) blocks are similar to iPACK blocks. Local anesthetic is injected at the medial epicondyle of the femur under ultrasound guidance. The anesthetic then spreads along fascial planes to the posterior capsule. Spread of anesthesia to the sciatic nerve is expected to have a lower incidence than the iPACK block.
- Posterior capsule infiltration. LIA injections can be used for posterior infiltration. Care should be used to avoid sciatic innervation. One study calls into question the benefit of posterior capsule infiltration and reports it is not necessary [30].

Anesthesia Adjuncts for Pain Control

- Ketamine Drip: Data on the efficacy and safety of ketamine in TJA are contradictory, and concern about side effects including hallucination and over sedation have limited its use. A recent study concluded that ketamine may not provide much additional benefit for pain control in knee arthroplasty [31].
- Lidocaine Drip: Lidocaine has been utilized in ERAS protocols for open abdominal procedures. There is a paucity of studies for TJA. Current clinical trials may help determine its usefulness in the outpatient setting [46].
- Liposomal Bupivacaine: The efficacy of liposomal bupivacaine in TJA relative to its substantially increased cost compared to generic anesthetics has been controversial. A Cochrane Database Systematic Review of randomized, double-blind, placebo- or active-controlled clinical trials of elective surgeries (including knee arthroplasty) reported no superiority of surgical site infiltration with liposomal bupivacaine compared to bupivacaine hydrochloride [32].
- Cryoanalgesia: Cryoanalgesia or cryoneurolysis delivers cold temperature to selected nerves to block the transmission of pain signals to the brain. The anterior and lateral femoral cutaneous nerves as well as the infrapatellar branch of the saphenous nerve are targeted for knee pain. Research evidence is sparse but one multicenter, randomized, double-blind study reported decreased pain in patients with mild to moderate knee osteoarthritis compared to sham control treatment for up to 150 days [33]. Up to a 45% reduction in opioid consumption over a 12 week postoperative period has been reported [34].
- Cooled Radiofrequency Treatment: Liquid-cooled thermal ablation of nerves has been studied for postoperative total knee pain. The superolateral, superomedial, and inferomedial genicular nerves are the target of this procedure. It has been shown to have positive pain control results for patients who are not candidates

for surgery or do not wish to have total knee surgery. It has not been shown to decrease opioid consumption post-knee arthroplasty [35].

Fluid Management

Fluid management is an important aspect of anesthesia for TJA. Too little fluid can possibly lead to acute kidney injury and too much fluid can contribute to postoperative urinary retention [36]. Classically, fluid management was based on the estimation of preoperative fluid deficits prior to anesthesia, maintenance requirements during surgery, and fluid losses during surgery. The 4/2/1 rule was used in this setting—4 mL/kg/h for the first 10 kg of body weight; 2 mL/kg/h for the next 10 kg of weight; and 1 mL/kg/h of body weight over 20 kg. This formula was used both for the amount of time the patient was NPO (nil per os) as well as for maintenance during the case.

Modern fluid management techniques focus on goal-directed therapy. Fluid interventions should be directed at a clinical variable that will optimize a patient's fluid status (e.g., stroke volume, respiratory variation). It is difficult to determine stroke volume or respiratory variation during TJA without invasive monitoring. However, blood pressure and possibly variation of pulse oximeter amplitude may give clinical indications of the need for intraoperative fluid. If a spinal is performed, a fluid bolus preoperatively is warranted. In general, more than two liters of crystalloid fluid (including the initial fluid bolus) is rarely needed if intraoperative blood loss falls within the normal range [37]. ERAS society recommendations state "It is recommended that intravenous fluids should be used judiciously and postoperative intravenous fluids discouraged in favor of early oral intake." [3].

Blood Loss

Tranexamic acid has been used extensively in TJA and has shown to decrease blood loss. It is a synthetic lysine analog that reversibly binds to the lysine receptor sites on plasminogen inhibiting the conversion of plasminogen to plasmin. Multiple studies have shown its safety profile. A clinical practice guide endorsed by both the American Academy of Hip and Knee Surgeons and the American Society of Regional Anesthesia and Pain Medicine is available [38].

Intraoperative Treatment of Nausea

Ondansetron and Dexamethasone are both effective for postoperative nausea. Female gender post-puberty, nonsmoking status, history of postoperative nausea and vomiting (PONV) or motion sickness, increasing duration of surgery, and use of volatile anesthetics, nitrous oxide, large-dose neostigmine, or intraoperative or postoperative opioids are well established PONV risk factors [39].

Postoperatively

Pain Management

Scheduled pain assessments should be performed prior to discharge. Typical scales include numerical rating scales which use numbers such as 0 = no pain to 10 = extreme pain, visual analog scales where patients mark the place on a scale corresponding to their pain level, and categorical scales where response options such as none, mild, moderate, and severe are used to communicate pain. Pain control protocols should be developed. Some programs advocate utilizing as little opioids as possible while others use opioids to help control moderate to severe pain. Opioids should be used sparingly if possible, but their use is appropriate for uncontrolled pain.

Intractable postoperative pain (i.e., pain unrelieved by modest doses of opioid medication) is rare. For hip arthroplasty patients with intractable pain, a rescue lateral femoral cutaneous nerve block should be considered. For knee arthroplasty patients with intractable anterior pain, an anterior femoral cutaneous nerve block may help. For lateral pain, a vastus lateralis nerve block may help. For posterior pain, a SPANK block can be used if no other posterior blocks have been performed.

Nausea and Vomiting

Pro re nata (PRN) orders for postoperative nausea typically include ondansetron and possibly promethazine or prochlorperazine. There is evidence that essential oils also are effective [40, 41].

Urinary Retention

Acute postoperative urinary retention (POUR) is a significant barrier to outpatient TJA as it can result in pathologic bladder distention and injury, urinary tract infection (with possible hematogenous periprosthetic infection), and catheterization-related complications. The incidence of acute POUR following TJA has been documented to range from 0 to 75%, varying based on the perioperative practices of TJA programs; characteristics of study populations; and definitions, measurement, and treatment methods for acute urinary retention [42]. High rates of POUR underscore the need for defined criteria and an established treatment plan. Most successful programs have an incidence below 5% [43]. Oliguria and acute kidney injury also are significant concerns.

While it is understood that POUR is defined by residual urine in the bladder 4 h after surgery, clinical criteria for the diagnosis of POUR (and commencement of catheterization treatment) are more arbitrary and variable. Although there are no TJA-specific guidelines, many surgeons use the adult urinary bladder capacity of 400–600 mL within 2–8 h of surgery as the threshold for intermittent catheterization [44]. A randomized controlled trial examining catheterization thresholds following fast-track TJA observed a significant reduction in postoperative catheterization from 32% when a 500 mL threshold was applied to 13% when an 800 mL threshold was used with no attendant increase in urological complications [45]. Clinical criteria and treatment protocols for POUR at our institution, resulting in a 3.9% incidence of POUR in same-day discharge patients, [43] are provided in Appendix 1.

Sample Outpatient TJA Anesthesia Protocol

The Indiana University Health Saxony Hip and Knee Center has safely performed 479 outpatient hip and knee arthroplasty procedures between September 2014 and November 2019. There have been no deaths. Data for cases performed by the end of July 2018 indicate an all-cause 90-day readmission rate of 3.7% (6 patients). Readmission reasons included atrial fibrillation, transient ischemic attack, superficial joint infection, deep joint infection, venous thromboembolism, and urinary tract infection. Medical risk stratification for outpatient selection [1, 2] and the standardized multimodal perioperative pain protocols provided in Appendix 2 have provided the foundation for us to safely provide outpatient TJA.

Appendix 1: Indiana University Health Saxony hip and Knee Center Call Orders for Postoperative Urinary Retention

Criterion for Oliguria Indication[1]

- Urine production less than 300 mL per 8 h shift
- Equates to 37.5 mL/h of urine production (300 mL/8 h)

Post-Anesthetic Care Unit documents time of last void prior to surgery.

Patients are asked to void in the 2–3 h postsurgical time frame. If unable, a bladder scan is performed.

- Scan >399: I/O catheterization is performed. Patient is then asked again to void after an additional 2 h and the process recurs until the patient is able to void.
- Scan <400: Pt is asked to void after another hour. If still unable to void then I/O catheterization is performed. Patients are then asked to void again after another 2 h and the process recurs until able to void. If the initial bladder scan shows less than 37.5 mL/h urine production since arrival then a bolus of 500 mL IV crystalloid is given.

Appendix 2: Indiana University Health Saxony hip and Knee Center Multimodal Perioperative Pain Protocol for Outpatient Arthroplasty

Prior to Arrival for Surgery

- Patients are encouraged to drink clear carbohydrate fluids up to 2 h before the scheduled arrival time. *Scheduled Arrival time* is emphasized rather than surgical time to maintain 2 h of NPO in case surgeries are running ahead of schedule.
- 24 h before arrival time, begin 1000 mg acetaminophen TID

Preoperative Unit

Unless contraindicated patients are given:

- Ondansetron 4 mg IV push
- Gabapentin 300 mg po
- Oxycodone ER 20 mg po

[1] Protocol pertains to patients without an indwelling catheter.

- Famotidine 20 mg po
- Acetaminophen 1000 mg
- Celecoxib 400 mg po (if renally appropriate and not allergic)
- Hydroxizine 25 mg po
- Pantoprazole 40 mg
- Kefzol IV weight appropriate or appropriate substitute

Fluid bolus 1 L crystalloid as appropriate.

Primary hip and knee patients are not catheterized. They are asked to urinate approximately 15 min prior to transfer to the operating room.

Intraoperatively

Primary Hips

- Spinal with Mepivacaine 1.5% approximately 37.5 mg but no more than 45 mg and 25 μg Fentanyl
- General with LMA or ETT as appropriate and as little inhaled agent as needed or TIVA
- Do not over-sedate patient with large doses of Midazolam in preparation for spinal administration. Patients need to be able to participate in physical therapy a few hours after surgery.
- If spinal appears to be wearing off before the procedure is completed (signs of increased respirations, etc.), a small dose of fentanyl, morphine, or dilaudid is given at the anesthesiologist's discretion.
- 1 g IV tranexamic acid after anesthesia induction and 1 g IV at closing
- Unless contraindicated patients receive approximately 2 L IV crystalloid including the preoperative bolus
- Ondansetron and/or Reglan or Compazine for nausea prophylaxis

Primary Knees

- Spinal with Mepivacaine 1.5% approximately 37.5 mg but no more than 45 mg and 25 μg Fentanyl
- General with LMA or ETT as appropriate and as little inhaled agent as needed or TIVA
- Do not over-sedate patient with large doses of Midazolam in preparation for spinal administration. Patients need to be able to participate in physical therapy a few hours after surgery.
- If the spinal appears to be wearing off before the procedure is completed (signs of increased respirations, etc.), a small dose of fentanyl, morphine, or dilaudid is given at the anesthesiologist's discretion.
- 15–20 mL ropivacaine 0.5% with 4 mg of dexamethasone deposited in distal adductor canal.

- Periarticular injection with ropivacaine 200 mg, clonidine 80 μg, epinephrine 0.5 mg in 100 mL.
- 1 g IV TXA after anesthesia induction and 1 g IV at closing
- Unless contraindicated patients receive approximately 2 L IV crystalloid including the preoperative bolus
- Ondansetron and/or Reglan or Compazine for nausea prophylaxis

Post-Anesthetic Care Unit

- Cold therapy
- PRN pain medications based on patient pain rating:
  - Tramadol 50 mg Q4 prn
  - Oxycodone IR 5 Q4 prn
  - Oxycodone IR 10 Q4 prn
  - Dilaudid 0.5 mg IV Q2 prn
  - Kefzol IV or appropriate substitute (must be 8 h after preoperative dose)
  - Ondansetron 4 mg IV prn
  - Prochlorperazine 10 mg IV prn
  - Diphenhydramine 12.5 mg prn
- Physical therapy evaluation
- Occupational therapy evaluation for hip patients and all patients with BMI ≥ 35

Discharge Medications and Orders

- Acetaminophen 1000 mg TID
- Oxycodone ER 10 mg Q12 x 5 days
- Oxycodone IR 10 mg 1/2–1 tab q4H prn
- Cefadroxil 500 mg BID x 7 days
- Omeprazole 20 mg daily
- ASA 81 mg BID
- Celecoxib 200 mg BID
- Gabapentin 300 mg BID
- Docusate-Senna
- Miralax
- Cold therapy
- Elevation

  In-home or outpatient physical therapy for knees only

References

1. Meneghini RM, et al. Safe selection of outpatient joint arthroplasty patients with medical risk stratification: the "outpatient arthroplasty risk assessment score". J Arthroplast. 2017;32(8):2325–31.
2. Ziemba-Davis M, Caccavallo P, Meneghini RM. Outpatient joint arthroplasty-patient selection: update on the outpatient arthroplasty risk assessment score. J Arthroplast. 2019;34(7s):S40–3.

3. Wainwright TW, et al. Consensus statement for perioperative care in total hip replacement and total knee replacement surgery: enhanced recovery after surgery (ERAS®) society recommendations. Acta Orthop. 2020;91(1):3–19.
4. Vanegas H, Vazquez E, Tortorici V. NSAIDs, opioids, cannabinoids and the control of pain by the central nervous system. Pharmaceuticals (Basel). 2010;3(5):1335–47.
5. Flake ZA, Scalley RD, Bailey AG. Practical selection of antiemetics. Am Fam Physician. 2004;69(5):1169–74.
6. Godshaw BM, et al. The effects of Peri-operative dexamethasone on patients undergoing total hip or knee arthroplasty: is it safe for diabetics? J Arthroplast. 2019;34(4):645–9.
7. Wasfie T, et al. Effect of intra-operative single dose of dexamethasone for control of post-operative nausea and vomiting on the control of glucose levels in diabetic patients. Am J Surg. 2018;215(3):488–90.
8. Honarmand A, et al. Prophylactic antiemetic effects of midazolam, ondansetron, and their combination after middle ear surgery. J Res Pharm Pract. 2016;5(1):16–21.
9. Pugely AJ, et al. Differences in short-term complications between spinal and general anesthesia for primary total knee arthroplasty. J Bone Joint Surg Am. 2013;95(3):193–9.
10. Matsen Ko L, Chen AF. Spinal anesthesia: the new gold standard for total joint arthroplasty? Ann Transl Med. 2015;3(12):162.
11. Fleisher LA, et al. 2014 ACC/AHA guideline on perioperative cardiovascular evaluation and management of patients undergoing noncardiac surgery: a report of the American College of Cardiology/American Heart Association task force on practice guidelines. J Am Coll Cardiol. 2014;64(22):e77–137.
12. Frisch NB, et al. Single-dose lidocaine spinal anesthesia in hip and knee arthroplasty. Arthroplast Today. 2018;4(2):236–9.
13. Ben-David B, et al. A comparison of minidose lidocaine-fentanyl and conventional-dose lidocaine spinal anesthesia. Anesth Analg. 2000;91(4):865–70.
14. Korhonen AM, et al. Intrathecal hyperbaric bupivacaine 3 mg + fentanyl 10 microg for outpatient knee arthroscopy with tourniquet. Acta Anaesthesiol Scand. 2003;47(3):342–6.
15. Horlocker, T.T., et al., Regional anesthesia in the patient receiving antithrombotic or thrombolytic therapy: American society of regional anesthesia and pain medicine evidence-based guidelines *(Fourth Edition)*. Reg Anesth Pain Med, 2018. 43(3): p. 263–309.
16. Anesthesiologists, A.S.o. Continuum of depth of sedation: definition of general anesthesia and levels of sedation/analgesia. 10/15/2014 [cited 2019 11/01/2019]. continuum-of-depth-of-sedation-definition-of-general-anesthesia-and-levels-of-sedationanalgesia.
17. Birnbaum K, et al. The sensory innervation of the hip joint--an anatomical study. Surg Radiol Anat. 1997;19(6):371–5.
18. Zhang XY, Ma JB. The efficacy of fascia iliaca compartment block for pain control after total hip arthroplasty: a meta-analysis. J Orthop Surg Res. 2019;14(1):33.
19. Stuart Green M, et al. Transmuscular quadratus Lumborum block reduces length of stay in patients receiving total hip arthroplasty. Anesth Pain Med. 2018;8(6):e80233.
20. Tulgar S, et al. Comparison of ultrasound-guided lumbar erector Spinae plane block and transmuscular quadratus lumborum block for postoperative analgesia in hip and proximal femur surgery: a prospective randomized feasibility study. Anesth Essays Res. 2018;12(4):825–31.
21. New York school of regional anesthesia: intra-articular and periarticular infiltration of local anesthetics. [cited 2019 November 1]. https://www.nysora.com/regional-anesthesia-for-specific-surgical-procedures/lower-extremity-regional-anesthesia-for-specific-surgical-procedures/anesthesia-and-analgesia-for-hip-procedures/intra-articular-periarticular-infiltration-local-anesthetics/.
22. Tran J, et al. Anatomical study of the innervation of anterior knee joint capsule: implication for image-guided intervention. Reg Anesth Pain Med. 2018;43(4):407–14.
23. Jaeger P, et al. Optimal volume of local anaesthetic for adductor canal block: using the continual reassessment method to estimate ED95. Br J Anaesth. 2015;115(6):920–6.

24. Zhang LK, et al. Single shot versus continuous technique adductor canal block for analgesia following total knee arthroplasty: a PRISMA-compliant meta-analysis. Medicine (Baltimore). 2019;98(20):e15539.
25. Elkassabany NM, et al. A prospective randomized open-label study of single injection versus continuous adductor canal block for postoperative analgesia after total knee arthroplasty. Bone Joint J. 2019;101-b(3):340–7.
26. Yuenyongviwat V, et al. Periarticular injection with bupivacaine for postoperative pain control in total knee replacement: a prospective randomized double-blind controlled trial. Adv Orthop. 2012;2012:107309.
27. Tsukada S, et al. Early stage periarticular injection during total knee arthroplasty may provide a better postoperative pain relief than late-stage periarticular injection: a randomized-controlled trial. Knee Surg Sports Traumatol Arthrosc. 2019;27(4):1124–31.
28. Grosso MJ, et al. Adductor Canal block compared with periarticular bupivacaine injection for total knee arthroplasty: a prospective randomized trial. J Bone Joint Surg Am. 2018;100(13):1141–6.
29. Kim DH, et al. Addition of infiltration between the popliteal artery and the capsule of the posterior knee and adductor canal block to periarticular injection enhances postoperative pain control in total knee arthroplasty: a randomized controlled trial. Anesth Analg. 2019;129(2):526–35.
30. Pinsornsak P, Nangnual S, Boontanapibul K. Multimodal infiltration of local anaesthetic in total knee arthroplasty; is posterior capsular infiltration worth the risk? A prospective, double-blind, randomised controlled trial. Bone Joint J. 2017;99-b(4):483–8.
31. Tan TL, et al. Intraoperative ketamine in Total knee arthroplasty does not decrease pain and narcotic consumption: a prospective randomized controlled trial. J Arthroplast. 2019;34(8):1640–5.
32. Hamilton TW, et al. Liposomal bupivacaine infiltration at the surgical site for the management of postoperative pain. Cochrane Database Syst Rev. 2017;2:Cd011419.
33. Radnovich R, et al. Cryoneurolysis to treat the pain and symptoms of knee osteoarthritis: a multicenter, randomized, double-blind, sham-controlled trial. Osteoarthr Cartil. 2017;25(8):1247–56.
34. Dasa V, et al. Percutaneous freezing of sensory nerves prior to total knee arthroplasty. Knee. 2016;23(3):523–8.
35. Walega D, et al. Radiofrequency ablation of genicular nerves prior to total knee replacement has no effect on postoperative pain outcomes: a prospective randomized sham-controlled trial with 6-month follow-up. Reg Anesth Pain Med. 2019;44(6):646–51.
36. Halawi MJ, et al. The Most significant risk factors for urinary retention in fast-track Total joint arthroplasty are iatrogenic. J Arthroplast. 2019;34(1):136–9.
37. Forget P, Lois F, de Kock M. Goal-directed fluid management based on the pulse oximeter-derived pleth variability index reduces lactate levels and improves fluid management. Anesth Analg. 2010;111(4):910–4.
38. Fillingham YA, et al. Tranexamic acid in total joint arthroplasty: the endorsed clinical practice guides of the American Association of hip and knee surgeons, American Society of regional anesthesia and pain medicine, American Academy of orthopaedic surgeons, hip society, and knee society. Reg Anesth Pain Med. 2019;44(1):7–11.
39. Gan TJ. Risk factors for postoperative nausea and vomiting. Anesth Analg. 2006;102(6):1884–98.
40. Fearrington MA, Qualls BW, Carey MG. Essential oils to reduce postoperative nausea and vomiting. J Perianesth Nurs. 2019;34(5):1047–53.
41. Hunt R, et al. Aromatherapy as treatment for postoperative nausea: a randomized trial. Anesth Analg. 2013;117(3):597–604.
42. Balderi T, Carli F. Urinary retention after total hip and knee arthroplasty. Minerva Anestesiol. 2010;76(2):120–30.
43. Ziemba-Davis M, et al. Identifiable risk factors to minimize postoperative urinary retention in modern outpatient rapid recovery Total joint arthroplasty. J Arthroplast. 2019;34(7s):S343–7.

44. Baldini G, et al. Postoperative urinary retention: anesthetic and perioperative considerations. Anesthesiology. 2009;110(5):1139–57.
45. Bjerregaard LS, et al. Postoperative urinary catheterization thresholds of 500 versus 800 mL after fast-track total hip and knee arthroplasty: a randomized, open-label, controlled trial. Anesthesiology. 2016;124(6):1256–64. https://pubs.asahq.org/anesthesiology/article/124/6/1256/14502/Postoperative-Urinary-Catheterization-Thresholds.

Chapter 8
Threats to Same Day Discharge: Prevention and Management

Charles P. Hannon, Parag D. Patel, and Craig J. Della Valle

Introduction

Historically, primary total joint arthroplasty (TJA) was associated with long inpatient hospital stays, extended postoperative recoveries, and significant patient morbidity. However, over the past 20 years, substantial advances have safely and effectively shifted TJA from an inpatient-only procedure to an outpatient procedure in properly selected patients [1–5].

The success of an outpatient TJA program is built upon appropriate patient selection, preoperative optimization, and patient education. In their review of 7747 TJAs discharged the same day, Sher et al. identified younger patients, patients with fewer comorbidities, and patients with lower body mass index as more likely to be safely discharged home [6]. For a majority of these carefully selected patients, outpatient TJA is very effective. Rates of severe adverse events after same day TJA have been reported as low as 1.3% [6]. However, there are challenges that occur in the outpatient setting that can delay discharge. Fraser et al., in their review of 106 patients preselected for same day discharge, found that 85% successfully met same day discharge criteria [7]. The most common medical reasons for not meeting discharge criteria included dizziness or hypotension, failure to clear physical therapy, urinary retention, and pain management. Patient preference was also a frequent reason for delayed discharge. In these instances, patients cleared medical and physical therapy

C. P. Hannon · C. J. Della Valle (✉)
Adult Reconstruction Division, Department of Orthopaedic Surgery, Rush University Medical Center, Chicago, IL, USA
e-mail: craig.dellavalle@rushortho.com

P. D. Patel
Department of Anesthesiology, Rush University Medical Center, Chicago, IL, USA

Rush Oakbrook Surgery Center, Oak Brook, IL, USA

R. M. Meneghini, L. T. Buller (eds.), *Outpatient Hip and Knee Replacement*,
https://doi.org/10.1007/978-3-031-27037-6_8

discharge criteria but preferred to stay overnight. Setting patient expectations through preoperative education and providing reassurance throughout the perioperative period is critical to helping mitigate this change in patient preference. However, medical complications still occur and threaten discharge. In this chapter, we review the most common threats to discharge in outpatient TJA and provide practical clinical advice on how to manage these complications.

Poor Pain Control

The key to addressing increased pain after TJA is prevention. Historically, opioids were the cornerstone of pain control after TJA. However, increased attention to opioids in light of today's epidemic has highlighted their adverse effects including sedation, respiratory depression, nausea, vomiting, urinary retention, and dependence. As a result, multimodal analgesia has evolved to be the standard of care in outpatient TJA [8].

As discussed in Chap. 5, the goal of multimodal analgesia is to give several analgesic medications at different time points that target different pain pathways [9]. Several studies have demonstrated that multimodal analgesia is associated with improved pain control, more rapid recovery, and shorter hospitalizations [10, 11]. Our multimodal regimen begins in the preoperative holding area with preemptive administration of oral acetaminophen, celecoxib, and pregabalin. The goal of preemptive medications is to blunt the peripheral and central nervous systems' response to tissue injury induced during surgery [12].

In the outpatient setting, we utilize a short acting spinal anesthetic for our hip surgeries to allow for rapid return of motor and sensory function. For patients undergoing knee surgery, we have successfully used both short acting spinal and general anesthesia, combined with an adductor canal block [13]. While neuraxial anesthetics have generally been preferred historically, we have found that general anesthesia can work very well for healthier patients as it minimizes the risks of many threats to discharge including urinary retention and delayed return of motor function. Intraoperatively, we use a periarticular injection that includes ropivacaine, epinephrine, ketorolac, and clonidine, which has been shown to further reduce pain and opioid consumption following TJA [13]. Patients also receive 15 mg of intravenous ketorolac and dexamethasone. Postoperatively, patients receive 1 g of acetaminophen every 8 h, 200 mg of celecoxib every 12 h, and 200 mg of gabapentin every 8 h. Tramadol is also given to patients as a scheduled medication in the early postoperative period, but it is later used as the first breakthrough pain medication. Oxycodone immediate release is used as a "last resort" breakthrough pain medication.

For the vast majority of patients, we have found that the multimodal regimen above is successful in adequately controlling pain postoperatively. However, some patients may have postoperative pain that is more challenging to control. In these cases, it is very helpful to work closely with the anesthesia and nursing staff to "troubleshoot" the situation and determine the most appropriate course of action. In knee patients with pain that is refractory to our standard regimen, we have found that the most common cause is an adductor canal block that is ineffective. In this situation, we will oftentimes consider having the anesthesia provider administer a femoral nerve block. It is important to recognize that femoral nerve blocks, while typically quite effective, are associated with quadriceps weakness and as such the patient is placed in a knee immobilizer for 48 h postoperatively until quadriceps function returns [14, 15]. In addition, we educate the patient and their family on the risk of falls and encourage the use of an appropriate assistive device. For patients with pain that is challenging to manage following hip surgery, we have had some success with an iliofascial block administered by anesthesia; however, the results are not as predictable. Intravenous opioid medications are used only as a last resort. In these situations, it is always imperative to ensure that the neurovascular status of the extremity is intact and that increased pain is not associated with phenomena such as a compartment syndrome. Rarely, inpatient admission is required for pain that cannot be adequately controlled.

Urinary Retention

Postoperative urinary retention (POUR) following outpatient TJA is one of the most common threats to early discharge. Rates of POUR have been identified as high as 3.9% for outpatient TJA patients [16]. In a review of 685 primary TJA discharged the same day or day after surgery Ziemba-Davis et al. identified male gender, a history of urinary retention, the use of rocuronium, glycopyrrolate, neostigmine, fentanyl spinal, and the absence of an indwelling urethral catheter as risk factors for POUR. Interestingly, male patients who received anticholinergics and cholinesterase inhibitors intraoperatively had a 31% increased rate of POUR. Several other studies have identified spinal anesthetics, as well as increased fluids (> 2 L) administered intraoperatively as risk factors for POUR [17, 18].

Given the high risk of POUR as a barrier to early discharge, it is prudent to quickly screen patients for risk factors for POUR and either perform their procedures as an inpatient or get a urological consult preoperatively. Patients who are identified as high risk for POUR are typically scheduled earlier in the day. To reduce the incidence of POUR, we encourage our anesthesiologists to avoid opioids, anticholinergics, and cholinesterase inhibitors, especially in male patients with a history of urinary retention. As stated above, for some patients a general anesthetic may be preferred, as well, to lower the risk. In the PACU, we encourage patients to hydrate with oral fluids. If patients are unable to void postoperatively, we encourage ambulation. If after approximately 4 h the patient is still unable to void, we use a bladder scanner to assess how much urine is in the bladder. If there is less than 400mL of urine in the bladder, we continue to encourage hydration and ambulation. However, if there is greater than 400mL we straight catheterize the patient. At this point, the patient must be carefully educated that if they do not start to void normally, they must either come back to the surgical facility for a repeat bladder scan, go see their primary care physician or present to an emergency department; careful and frequent follow-up with the patient by telephone is recommended. The other alternative is to place a foley catheter and discharge the patient home and then have the patient see their primary care physician or urologist for catheter removal and reassessment.

Hypotension and Tachycardia

Hypotension and tachycardia used to be common after TJA due to increased blood loss in surgery. However, with the routine use of tranexamic acid, perioperative blood loss has been dramatically reduced. Tranexamic acid acts as an anti-fibrinolytic agent by competitively inhibiting the conversion of plasminogen to plasmin. The American Association of Hip and Knee Surgeons clinical practice guideline recommends tranexamic acid be given routinely in TJA because of the decreased blood loss and transfusion rates when compared to placebo [19]. This has been widely adopted and is now the standard of care in TJA, but the optimal dosing and route of administration remain debated [20]. At our ambulatory surgery centers, we administer 1950 mg of tranexamic orally in the preoperative area prior to the procedure.

The risk of hypotension postoperatively is an additional reason we prefer to use general anesthesia in the outpatient setting when otherwise safe for the patient. We also encourage hydration preoperatively with clear liquids allowed for up to 4 h prior to the procedure. Patients who are on angiotensin-converting enzyme (ACE) inhibitors or angiotensin receptor blockers (ARB) for hypertension are instructed to not take these medications the morning of surgery as these can exacerbate hypotension intraoperatively. Postoperatively, if a patient has persistent hypotension we encourage oral fluid intake. If the patient is not able to tolerate oral liquids we work closely with our anesthesia colleagues to address the hypotension. We typically first administer a 500–1000 mL intravenous fluid bolus in the PACU to see how the patient responds. We closely monitor the patient in the PACU. If there is a concern for other medical causes of hypotension besides hypovolemia, we immediately contact an internal medicine colleague to assist with management. In the outpatient setting, these providers are not on site, but they are readily available by phone at our academic tertiary care center to provide recommendations. If there is any concern, we transfer the patient to an emergency department or can monitor the patient overnight as all of our ambulatory surgical centers have 23 h observation capabilities. Consideration should be made for this potential complication and a plan developed depending on your outpatient center's capacity.

Hypoxia

Hypoxia postoperatively is uncommon after outpatient TJA in properly selected patients. At our institution, patients at increased risk for hypoxia (e.g., obstructive sleep apnea, chronic obstructive pulmonary disease) are not offered outpatient surgery to specifically prevent this postoperative complication or are scheduled early in the day. Patients with obstructive sleep apnea (OSA) are 2–4 times more likely to develop a medical complication after TJA compared to patients without OSA [21]. Many patients with OSA are undiagnosed and thus we work closely with our internal medicine colleagues to be sure that OSA is screened for during medical clearance. Grau et al. found in their study of 7658 TJA that instituting a pulmonary screening questionnaire and intervention protocol resulted in a 63-fold reduction in pulmonary complications after TJA [14].

Another advantage of our multimodal analgesia protocol that limits opioids is that it, too, helps prevent hypoxia postoperatively. However, if a patient presents with hypoxia in the PACU we begin by administering oxygen via nasal cannula. The patient's oxygen saturation and heart rate are then continually monitored. As with several of the other threats to discharge, we work closely with our anesthesia colleagues to address this situation. We have portable X-ray available at our ambulatory surgical centers and can get an anteroposterior chest radiograph if needed. We encourage patients with hypoxia to utilize the incentive spirometer, as well. Often this hypoxia is seen early in the PACU after surgery and is associated with sedation from anesthesia or opioid use. If opioid-induced respiratory depression is suspected we have naloxone available. The patient is then closely monitored after the procedure and in most cases resolves. However, if the hypoxia persists we consult our internal medicine colleagues. If there is any concern, we transfer the patient to an emergency department or can monitor the patient overnight.

Nausea and Vomiting

Nausea and vomiting are common after any surgical procedure. As with several of the threats to discharge discussed previously, prevention is key. We encourage patients to hydrate up to 4 h prior to surgery with clear liquids. Throughout the patient's stay, we limit the use of opioids, which are associated with high rates of nausea and vomiting. Intraoperatively, patients receive 10 mg of dexamethasone, which decreases rates of nausea and vomiting after surgery. Tammachote et al. found that patients who received 0.15 mg/kg of IV dexamethasone had better postoperative pain relief and lower rates of nausea and vomiting compared to patients who received a saline placebo.[15]. In addition, propofol, which is used for sedation during neuraxial anesthesia, has a good antiemetic effect [22]. Propofol can also be utilized as a component of general anesthesia to limit the use of anesthetic gasses that increase the risk of postoperative nausea and vomiting.

If a patient has persistent nausea after surgery, we initially give IV ondansetron 4 mg every 4 h. We encourage hydration orally if the patient can tolerate oral intake. If they cannot tolerate oral fluids we give intravenous fluids. If nausea persists after ondansetron we give IV metoclopramide 10 mg. Typically, hydration and these medications resolve nausea. Intramuscular ephedrine can also be used off-label to treat nausea and vomiting and is reserved for refractory cases. While the mechanism is not well understood, the sympathomimetic properties of ephedrine likely help with lethargy, dizziness, and nausea. Patients who are concerned with nausea after discharge are prescribed oral dissolving tablets of ondansetron 4 mg to take every 8 h as needed.

Unable to Safely Meet Physical Therapy Discharge Criteria

Proper patient selection and effective pain control are critical to ensuring that patients are able to meet same day physical therapy discharge criteria. Maximizing pain control as described above is important to ensure that patients are able to participate in physical therapy. The use of general anesthesia or a short acting spinal as well as an adductor canal block all minimize motor weakness that can inhibit participation in physical therapy. We encourage the use of assistive devices during physical therapy and have a physical therapist either on site or in an adjacent facility to ensure that patients can safely ambulate prior to discharge. We attempt to schedule patients preoperatively identified as potentially requiring additional therapy prior to discharge as the first or second case so that they can have two therapy sessions on the day of surgery. If a patient is still unable to meet discharge criteria, we have the patient stay overnight in our observation unit and meet with physical therapy in the morning.

Conclusion

Outpatient TJA is safe and effective for properly selected patients. While most patients are able to safely discharge the same day after their TJA, complications can occur after surgery that threatens to delay discharge. Dealing with these complications such as poor postoperative pain control and POUR can often be avoided with proper selection and multimodal analgesia that limits opioids. However, when these complications present after surgery, close care coordination with anesthesiology and, if needed, internal medicine can help safely and effectively mitigate these threats to discharge and allow patients to be discharged within 24 h. Patients with complications require close follow-up after discharge and should be educated on the importance of contacting their surgeon's team if any concerns or issues arise.

References

1. Parcells BW, Giacobbe D, Macknet D, Smith A, Schottenfeld M, Harwood DA, et al. Total joint arthroplasty in a stand-alone ambulatory surgical center: short-term outcomes. Orthopedics. 2016;39:223–8. https://doi.org/10.3928/01477447-20160419-06.

2. Goyal N, Chen AF, Padgett SE, Tan TL, Kheir MM, Hopper RH, et al. Otto Aufranc award: a multicenter, randomized study of outpatient versus inpatient total hip arthroplasty. Clin Orthop Relat Res. 2017;475:364–72. https://doi.org/10.1007/s11999-016-4915-z.
3. Berger RA, Sanders SA, Thill ES, Sporer SM, Valle C. Newer anesthesia and rehabilitation protocols enable outpatient hip replacement in selected patients. Clin Orthop Relat Res. 2009;467:1424–30. https://doi.org/10.1007/s11999-009-0741-x.
4. Basques BA, Tetreault MW, Valle CJ. Same-day discharge compared with inpatient hospitalization following hip and knee arthroplasty. J Bone Jt Surg. 2017;99:1969–77. https://doi.org/10.2106/jbjs.16.00739.
5. Hoffmann JD, Kusnezov NA, Dunn JC, Zarkadis NJ, Goodman GP, Berger RA. The shift to same-day outpatient joint arthroplasty: a systematic review. J Arthroplast. 2018;33:1265–74. https://doi.org/10.1016/j.arth.2017.11.027.
6. Sher A, Keswani A, Yao D, Anderson M, Koenig K, Moucha CS. Predictors of same-day discharge in primary total joint arthroplasty patients and risk factors for post-discharge complications. J Arthroplast. 2017;32:S150–S156.e1. https://doi.org/10.1016/j.arth.2016.12.017.
7. Fraser JF, Danoff JR, Manrique J, Reynolds MJ, Hozack WJ. Identifying reasons for failed same-day discharge following primary total hip arthroplasty. J Arthroplast. 2018;33:3624–8. https://doi.org/10.1016/j.arth.2018.08.003.
8. Hannon CP, Keating T, Lange JK, Ricciardi BF, Waddell BS, Valle CJ. Anesthesia and analgesia practices in total joint arthroplasty: a survey of the AAHKS membership. J Arthroplast. 2019;34(12):2872–7. https://doi.org/10.1016/j.arth.2019.06.055.
9. Kehlet H, Dahl JB. The value of "multimodal" or "balanced analgesia" in postoperative pain treatment. Anesth Analg. 1993;77:1048. https://doi.org/10.1213/00000539-199311000-00030.
10. Sah AP, Liang K, Sclafani JA. Optimal multimodal analgesia treatment recommendations for total joint arthroplasty. JBJS Rev. 2018;6:e7. https://doi.org/10.2106/jbjs.rvw.17.00137.
11. Golladay GJ, Balch KR, Dalury DF, Satpathy J, Jiranek WA. Oral multimodal analgesia for total joint arthroplasty. J Arthroplast. 2017;32:S69–73. https://doi.org/10.1016/j.arth.2017.05.002.
12. Kissin I. Preemptive analgesia: terminology and clinical relevance. Anesth Analg. 1994;79:809. https://doi.org/10.1213/00000539-199410000-00037.
13. Ma H-H, Chou T-F, Tsai S-W, Chen C-F, Wu P-K, Chen W-M. The efficacy of intraoperative periarticular injection in total hip arthroplasty: a systematic review and meta-analysis. Bmc Musculoskelet Di. 2019;20:269. https://doi.org/10.1186/s12891-019-2628-7.
14. Grau L, Orozco FR, Duque AF, Post Z, Fink B, Ong AC. A simple protocol to stratify pulmonary risk reduces complications after total joint arthroplasty. J Arthroplast. 2019;34:1233–9. https://doi.org/10.1016/j.arth.2019.01.048.
15. Tammachote N, Kanitnate S. Intravenous dexamethasone injection reduces pain from twelve to twenty-one hours after total knee arthroplasty: a double-blind randomized placebo controlled trial. J Arthroplast. 2019;35(2):394–400. https://doi.org/10.1016/j.arth.2019.09.002.
16. Ziemba-Davis M, Nielson M, Kraus K, Duncan N, Nayyar N, Meneghini MR. Identifiable risk factors to minimize postoperative urinary retention in modern outpatient rapid recovery total joint arthroplasty. J Arthroplast. 2019;34:S343–7. https://doi.org/10.1016/j.arth.2019.03.015.
17. Lawrie CM, Ong AC, Hernandez VH, Rosas S, Post ZD, Orozco FR. Incidence and risk factors for postoperative urinary retention in total hip arthroplasty performed under spinal anesthesia. J Arthroplast. 2017;32:3748–51. https://doi.org/10.1016/j.arth.2017.07.009.
18. Scholten R, Kremers K, van de Groes S, Somford DM, Koëter S. Incidence and risk factors of postoperative urinary retention and bladder catheterization in patients undergoing fast-track total joint arthroplasty: a prospective observational study on 371 patients. J Arthroplast. 2018;33:1546–51. https://doi.org/10.1016/j.arth.2017.12.001.
19. Fillingham YA, Ramkumar DB, Jevsevar DS, Yates AJ, Bini SA, Clarke HD, et al. Tranexamic acid use in Total joint arthroplasty: the clinical practice guidelines endorsed by the American Association of hip and knee surgeons, American Society of Regional Anesthesia and Pain Medicine, American Academy of Orthopaedic surgeons, hip society, and knee society. J Arthroplast. 2018;33:3065–9. https://doi.org/10.1016/j.arth.2018.08.002.

20. Abdel MP, Berry DJ. AAHKS symposium current practice trends in primary hip and knee arthroplasties among members of the American Association of hip and knee surgeons: an long-term update. J Arthroplast. 2019;34:S24–7. https://doi.org/10.1016/j.arth.2019.02.006.
21. Vakharia RM, Cohen-Levy W, Vakharia AM, Donnally C, Law T, Roche MW. Sleep apnea increases 90-day complications and cost following primary total joint arthroplasty. J Arthroplast. 2018;34:959–964.e1. https://doi.org/10.1016/j.arth.2018.12.018.
22. Chang C-C, Wong C-S. Postoperative nausea and vomiting free for all: a solution from propofol? Acta Anaesthesiol Taiwanica. 2017;54:106–7. https://doi.org/10.1016/j.aat.2016.12.002.

Chapter 9
Is there an Optimal Place for Outpatient TJA: Hospital, ASC, or "Other"?

William G. Hamilton, Roshan T. Melvani, and Agnes D. Cororaton

In recent years the use of outpatient total joint arthroplasty (TJA) has increased with advancements in perioperative protocols and refined anesthesia techniques. Outpatient TJA can be performed either in a full-service hospital within the hospital outpatient department (HOPD), or in a free-standing ambulatory surgery center (ASC). HOPDs are under financial control and usually owned by the hospital, and are often physically attached to the full-service hospital. Furthermore, any unit may be considered an HOPD if it has financial or administrative contracts with a hospital and is within 35 miles of the hospital [1]. ASCs are stand-alone facilities that operate with their own Medicare agreements and abide by the ASC Covered Procedures List dictated by Center for Medicare and Medicaid Services (CMS). Total knee arthroplasty (TKA) was removed from the inpatient-only (IPO) list in 2018, and as of January 2020 was added to the ASC covered procedure list. Also in January 2020, total hip arthroplasty (THA) was removed from the IPO list, but will still not be allowed to be performed in a free-standing ASC. Private insurers will usually allow these procedures to be performed in either an ASC or HOPD.

Patient Mindset

Most surgeons agree that one of the most important factors leading to a successful outpatient TJA is the patient's intention, conviction, and willingness to go home on the day of surgery. Currently, overnight stays are favored for patients or families that strongly prefer the sense of security they get from staying overnight in a facility. However, there is a growing acceptance and preference among patients to discharge

W. G. Hamilton (✉) · R. T. Melvani · A. D. Cororaton
Anderson Orthopaedic Research Institute, Alexandria, VA, USA
e-mail: agnesc@aori.org

R. M. Meneghini, L. T. Buller (eds.), *Outpatient Hip and Knee Replacement*,
https://doi.org/10.1007/978-3-031-27037-6_9

home on the day of surgery. The acceptance of outpatient TJA is likely influenced by the regional prevalence of same-day TJA.

It can be difficult to quantify this shifting mindset, and there is little published on the subject. Meneghini et al. reported on a questionnaire that was used on 110 consecutive patients scheduled for TJA. Three patients expected same day discharge, 17 expected one-night stay at the hospital, and 54 expected two or more nights at the hospital. Approximately half of the patients were aware of the outpatient TJA option, with 55.3% of men and 31.7% of women reporting that they were comfortable with outpatient TJA ($p = 0.03$). The majority believed that faster recovery and decreased likelihood of infection were advantages of outpatient TJA. Approximately half of the patients in the study felt ambulatory surgery centers were as safe as hospitals and believed that their individual home is the best place to recover from TJA [2].

Husted et al. investigated 50 patients (30 TKA, 20 THA) who had surgery at an ASC. Immediately after surgery, patients were then randomized to either recover in the ASC or transfer to recover in a hospital arthroplasty ward. Twenty-four out of twenty-five patients in the ASC group were discharged on the day of surgery (DOS) compared with 20/25 discharged on the DOS from the hospital ward ($p = 0.08$). All THA patients were discharged on the DOS and more TKA patients were discharged from the ASC (15/16) compared to the hospital (9/14) ($p = 0.04$). The authors offered several explanations that may have contributed to these differences. Those randomized to the hospital group stayed with other inpatients from different specialties, potentially influencing their state of mind. Also, patients in the hospital ward had regular beds which likely did not encourage easy mobilization, whereas ASC patients had recovery beds that mimicked sitting and standing positions. They also hypothesized that the staff influenced discharge, including a dedicated anesthesiologist who monitored and managed pain, nausea, and dizziness in the ASC compared to the hospital ward where this was not the case [3].

Kelly et al. investigated patient satisfaction among 174 TJA patients. Outpatients responded with more encouraging responses when asked about the staff's explanation of any prescription medications (outpatient = 91.4% vs. inpatient = 77.5%, $p = 0.026$), the staff's assistance with their pain management (98.3% vs. 88.0%, $p = 0.022$), discharge instructions (98.3% vs. 90.1%, $p = 0.05$), and the courtesy and respect from the nursing staff (100.0% vs. 92.2%, $p = 0.022$). Inpatients responded with less satisfaction when asked how prepared they felt for discharge home (8.9% vs. 0.0%, $p = 0.014$). The best responses in overall satisfaction with the facility (87.1% vs. 93.4%, $p = 0.204$) and overall experience (89.2% vs. 95.2%, $p = 0.177$) were similar between inpatients and outpatients, respectively. Inpatients in this study were older, heavier, and had higher Charlson comorbidity scores [4].

Differences in Cost

Studies have suggested that Medicare and individual patients can save on payments and out-of-pocket costs when procedures are performed in ASCs compared to HOPDs. The cost to CMS is typically lower when procedures are performed at an ASC, with one article reporting that the average ASC costs 53% of the amount paid to HOPD [1]. This same article reported that knee arthroscopy was $1005 at an ASC compared to $2098 at HOPD while knee arthroplasty was $5914 at an ASC compared to $9349 at HOPD. Medicare saved $2.3 billion with procedures done at an ASC in 2011 and is projected to save $57 billion in the next 10 years with procedures done at ASCs. Patient out-of-pocket costs for orthopedic procedures amount to approximately $251 at ASC compared to $524 for HOPD [1]. While out-of-network issues with insurance companies potentially add another layer of complexity to the cost that needs to be addressed in the future, data has shown that ASCs can accommodate cost-effective procedures.

Physicians who have financial ownership in an ASC are allowed by law to refer Medicare and Medicaid patients to their centers [5]. ASCs may be more responsive to physician control and allow for financial incentives that pave the way for direct accountability that may increase the quality of care.

Recommendations for Same Day Discharge

Effective same day discharge protocols require efficiency throughout the surgical process. Patients must be educated in the office setting to insure comfort with the concept of outpatient TJA. Ideally, centers should have efficient registration, patient preparation, and timely discharge post-procedure to reduce prolonged patient waiting times. Easily accessible locations with convenient parking improve patient satisfaction. It is helpful when nursing staff are accustomed to an efficient routine that helps prepare patients for surgery, including placing peripheral IVs, giving preoperative medications, and setting patient and family expectations. Anesthesia staff should collaborate with surgical staff and use proven protocols in a timely fashion to optimize outcomes. We favor the use of spinal anesthesia, but general anesthesia can be safely employed. The operating room team's preparation for setup and draping should be uniform, simple, and reproducible. Appropriate backup or revision equipment should be available to handle intraoperative complications [6].

In the recovery room, narcotic medications should be used judiciously to avoid over-medication that can lead to side effects of nausea and drowsiness. Anti-nausea medications should be given prophylactically. Soon after admission to the post-anesthesia care unit, patients can be transitioned from intravenous to oral fluids and medications in preparation for discharge. Discharge instructions should be simple and safe; providers should take the time to make sure that patients understand the instructions clearly. To qualify for discharge, patients must ambulate and safely meet discharge criteria. Avoiding safety events leading to readmission is of paramount importance. Occasionally an overnight stay is required, so screening for patients at higher risk for urinary retention, intractable pain or nausea, hypotension, transportation issues, or social issues can help prevent transfer to an inpatient facility. Performing higher risk cases in a facility that has overnight capability may be preferable.

Outcomes

While the literature comparing outcomes between these ASCs and HOPDs is preliminary and limited, early data indicates that these two settings have comparable patient outcomes. Careful patient selection is a factor in all of these reports leading to substantial selection bias. However, a few recent studies have studied this topic. One report performed a randomized study comparing 112 outpatient THAs discharged with 108 inpatient primary THAs. The study showed no differences in reoperations, hospital admissions without reoperation, emergency department visits without reoperation, or acute office visits between groups. Inclusion criteria in this study included age less than 75 years at the time of surgery, BMI < 40, opioid naïve, and no requirement for ambulatory assistance. The visual analog scale pain was comparable on the day of surgery (inpatient =2.5 vs. outpatient =3.3, $p = 0.12$), but was higher for outpatients on the first day after surgery (2.8 vs. 3.7, $p = 0.005$). Furthermore, there were no differences in the number of correspondences with the surgeon's office suggesting that outpatient THAs can be implemented without requiring increased work postoperatively for the surgeon's staff [7].

Sershon et al. evaluated 965 primary THAs who underwent same day discharge from either an ASC ($n = 335$) or from a HOPD ($n = 630$). The study demonstrated no increased complications regardless of the setting. Additionally, no differences were found between groups for 90-day complication rates (ASC = 3.9% vs. HOPD = 3.8%, $p = 0.48$), revision rates (0% vs. 0.3%, $p = 0.30$), all-cause reoperation rates (0.3% vs. 0.8%, $p = 0.35$), emergency department visits (0.9% vs. 0.3%, $p = 0.23$), or readmission rates (0.6% vs. 1.4%, $p = 0.25$) [8]. Another retrospective study compared 288 outpatient unicompartmental knee arthroplasties (UKA) performed in an ASC with 281 from HOPD. There was no difference in the overall 90-day complication rate (ASC = 4.2% vs. HOP = 6.4%, $p = 0.26$), day of surgery admission (0 vs. 0.4%, $p = 0.49$), emergency department visits less than 24 h after surgery (0.3% vs. 0.4%, $p = 1.0$), emergency department visits within 3 days of surgery (1.0% vs. 1.4%, $p = 0.72$), and readmissions in the first 90 days (1.7% vs. 2.8%, $p = 0.41$) between groups [9].

Conclusion

Outpatient TJA is a growing trend and surgeons should be familiar with all of the factors required for safely performing these procedures. While either the ASC or HOPD can be utilized for outpatient TJA, ASCs provide efficiency, physician autonomy, and potential cost savings. HOPDs may still be ideal for surgeons who are initiating the outpatient TJA process, as well as patients with risk factors that require a safety net in the event of a complication.Conflict of InterestAuthor WGH has part ownership of an ambulatory surgery center, receives research support from Biomet, receives IP royalties and research support and is a paid consultant and presenter for DePuy, A Johnson & Johnson Company, receives research support for Inova Health Care Services, and receives IP royalties and is a paid consultant for Total Joint Orthopaedics. Authors RM and ADC have nothing to disclose.

References

1. Tanaka, M. Ambulatory surgery centers versus hospital-based outpatient departments: what's the difference? AAOS Now 2019.
2. Meneghini RM, Ziemba-Davis M. Patient perceptions regarding outpatient hip and knee arthroplasties. J Arthroplast. 2017;32(9):2701–2705.e1. https://doi.org/10.1016/j.arth.2017.04.006.
3. Husted C, Gromov K, Hansen HK, Troelsen A, Kristensen BB, Husted H. Outpatient total hip or knee arthroplasty in ambulatory surgery center versus arthroplasty ward: a randomized controlled trial. Acta Orthop. 2019;4:1–9. https://doi.org/10.1080/17453674.2019.1686205.
4. Kelly MP, Calkins TE, Culvern C, Kogan M, Della Valle CJ. Inpatient versus outpatient hip and knee arthroplasty: which has higher patient satisfaction? J Arthroplast. 2018;33(11):3402–6. https://doi.org/10.1016/j.arth.2018.07.025.
5. Iglehart JK. The emergence of physician owned specialty hospitals. N Engl J Med. 2005;352(1):78–84.
6. Hamilton WG. Protocol development for outpatient Total joint arthroplasty. J Arthroplast. 2019;34(7S):S46–7. https://doi.org/10.1016/j.arth.2018.12.043.
7. Goyal N, Chen AF, Padgett SE, Tan TL, Kheir MM, Hopper RH Jr, Hamilton WG, Hozack WJ. Otto Aufranc award: a multicenter, randomized study of outpatient versus inpatient total hip arthroplasty. Clin Orthop Relat Res. 2017;475(2):364–72. https://doi.org/10.1007/s11999-016-4915-z.
8. Sershon RA, McDonald JF 3rd, Ho H, Goyal N, Hamilton WG. Outpatient total hip arthroplasty performed at an ambulatory surgery center vs hospital outpatient setting: complications, revisions, and readmissions. J Arthroplast. 2019;34(12):2861–5. https://doi.org/10.1016/j.arth.2019.07.032.
9. Cody JP, Pfefferle KJ, Ammeen DJ, Fricka KB. Is outpatient unicompartmental knee arthroplasty safe to perform at an ambulatory surgery center? A comparative study of early post-operative complications. J Arthroplast. 2018;33(3):673–6. https://doi.org/10.1016/j.arth.2017.10.007.

Chapter 10
Navigating the Limitations and Obstacles of TJA in a Free-Standing ASC

Nicholas B. Frisch and Richard A. Berger

Patient Selection

Choosing the right patient is critical to success in a free-standing ASC. An entire chapter of this book is devoted to selecting the right patient from a medical and safety standpoint, but its importance cannot be overstated. When performing a joint replacement in a hospital, those criteria are important, but if something is missed, you have options. If a patient does not do well for any reason after surgery, they can be admitted to observation units, to the floor for additional monitoring, or in some cases a surgical intensive care unit.

It is imperative to understand the capabilities of the particular ASC in which you operate. Each facility is different, both in terms of available accommodations, capacity, and staffing. Some facilities have the option of 23 h observation, while others do not. Some facilities may even be licensed for longer lengths of stay, while others may require transfer to a facility that can accommodate a higher level of care. Furthermore, there are typically dedicated rooms required for the patient that may need to meet certain requirements and also accommodate family or friends staying with them (Fig. 10.1). For those facilities that do have extended stay options, there will be an additional requirement for anesthesia provider coverage and on-call coverage. Additional coverage options can be logistically challenging and limited in capacity depending on the facility. Understanding how many overnight rooms are available to the patient and their family may impact

N. B. Frisch (✉)
Department of Orthopaedic Surgery, Ascension Providence Rochester Hospital, Rochester, MI, USA
e-mail: nick@gafrisch.com

R. A. Berger
Department of Orthopaedic Surgery, Rush University Medical Center, Chicago, IL, USA

R. M. Meneghini, L. T. Buller (eds.), *Outpatient Hip and Knee Replacement*,
https://doi.org/10.1007/978-3-031-27037-6_10

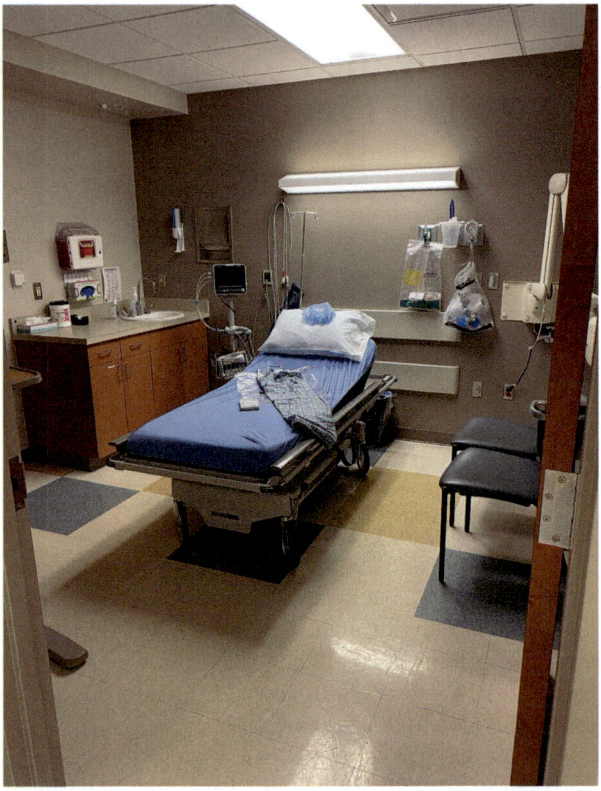

Fig. 10.1 Dedicated room for overnight stay and up to 23 h observation

which cases are boarded on which days and how many cases surgeons are comfortable doing on those days. There are different regulations around how long a patient can stay in an ASC. A protocol should be in place to ensure that there is a process for managing patient discharge prior to the 24 h time limit. To that point, surgeons need to know the options for transferring and what arrangements the ASC has in circumstances where this may become necessary. Specifically, whether they have a contract with an ambulance or transportation company to facilitate the transfer? Are you as a surgeon credentialed at the facility where your patient may be transferred? If not, do you have a colleague who can manage your patient upon transfer?

Choosing the right patient also encompasses surgical options. Instead of allowing their administrator, or the patient, to decide if a case goes to the ASC, surgeons should assess the patient's medical status, their need for special equipment, and the complexity of the case before offering the ASC as an option. Whether it is a unicompartmental knee arthroplasty that requires conversion to a total knee arthroplasty (TKA), a TKA that requires additional constraint, or a complex total hip arthroplasty that requires less frequently utilized implant options or specialized stems, the surgeon should assess whether each case is suitable for the ASC.

Space—A Different Frontier in an ASC

Part of the efficiency and cost-effectiveness of an ASC is the appropriate utilization of space. Each square foot of space has a value. The surgeon's experience in an ASC can usually be broken down into a relatively straightforward process. As a surgeon, think about what your steps are from the time you pull into the parking lot to the time you drive home. Most likely it resembles something like this:

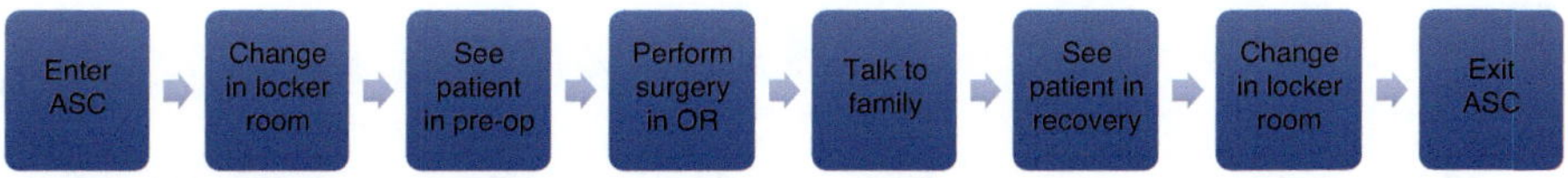

As such, the perception of space may be limited to those specific experiences and encounters. But from a facility design standpoint, space is significantly more sophisticated. While layout will inevitably vary between facilities, there are other critical functions that dictate a surgeon's ability to perform joint replacement at the ASC.

From a 10,000-foot view, it is first important to realize that space extends beyond the scope of the physical building. Parking ratios are calculated to ensure appropriate parking for patients, staff, and physicians. Depending on the location there may be other tenants in the building, or the ASC is part of a larger facility such as a mall or medical office building (MOB). Depending on the size of the ASC and the case mix (i.e., joints, spine, sports, etc.), the throughput may affect these ratios and will be calculated accordingly. The size of the waiting room is another example. How many chairs are needed for family members (what is the average number of people that accompany each patient)? To calculate these numbers requires predictive modeling for the number of patients in the preoperative area, the operating room, and the recovery room at one given time. During that time, family and friends will require adequate space to wait. Efficiently scheduling and managing that process will ensure that there is ample space and comfort without overcrowding, but not excessive space that could be repurposed to add more value to the center.

A common theme in ASCs is the cross-utilization of space. This is most commonly seen in the preoperative and recovery areas. Depending on the daily volume and case mix, earlier in the day the recovery area can be used similarly to the preoperative area to prepare patients for surgery. As the day progresses, the preoperative area can be transitioned to a recovery area. In contrast, most hospitals have separate dedicated preoperative and postoperative space that may or may not be in proximity to one another (Figs. 10.2 and 10.3). The ability to cross-utilize space is often planned during facility design so that the two areas are in close proximity to one another. This also affords the ability to cross-utilize staff so that nurses and staff can work together, using the same protocols in both the preoperative and recovery process. While staffing ratios will inevitably vary between facilities, this is a common practice and can have a positive impact on staff overhead.

When talking about the physical space of the ASC from an operating standpoint, there are several important considerations. Understanding the requirements

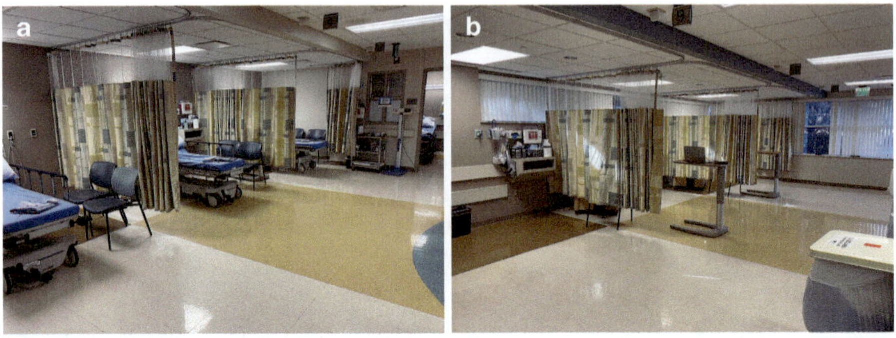

Fig. 10.2 Ambulatory surgery center (**a**) preoperative area and (**b**) recovery area. Although the images are not large enough to show the true layout, the preoperative and recovery areas are directly adjacent to one another for the purpose of cross-utilization as needed

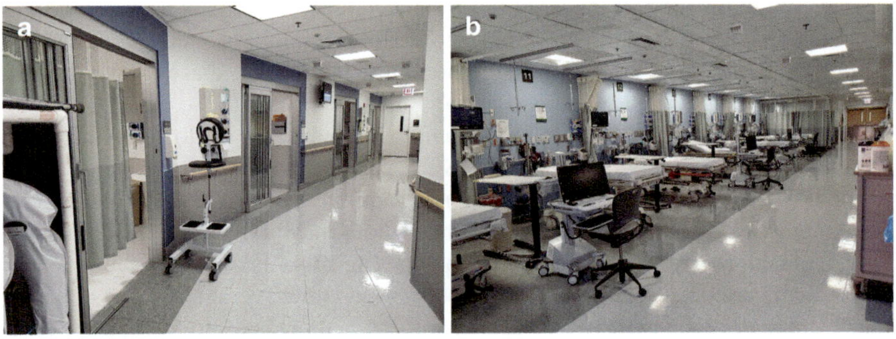

Fig. 10.3 Hospital (**a**) preoperative area and (**b**) recovery area. Note that the recovery picture represents only one pod of several at a larger hospital facility

necessary to perform certain procedures such as TJA will determine the necessary infrastructure and facility design. Focusing specifically on joint replacement, there are four main categories that must be considered: (1) Instruments, (2) Implants, (3) Disposable Goods, and (4) Sterile Processing. Storage of disposable goods requires careful inventory management. Given space limitations the overall quantity of goods stored is often far less than in hospitals. Leadership will closely monitor inventory and manage restocking and delivery in real time to accommodate the cases on the schedule, but ensure no overcrowding of storage space (Figs. 10.4 and 10.5).

The close management of inventory requires surgeons to be prepared not just for the procedure, but request any specialized equipment necessary in the event of an issue. For example, a patient may have unrecognized ligament laxity or there may be an intraoperative injury to the medial collateral ligament (MCL), which while rare has been reported to occur in 0.5–3% of TKA [1–4]. Either case would require additional implant requirements to address appropriately. There are many options,

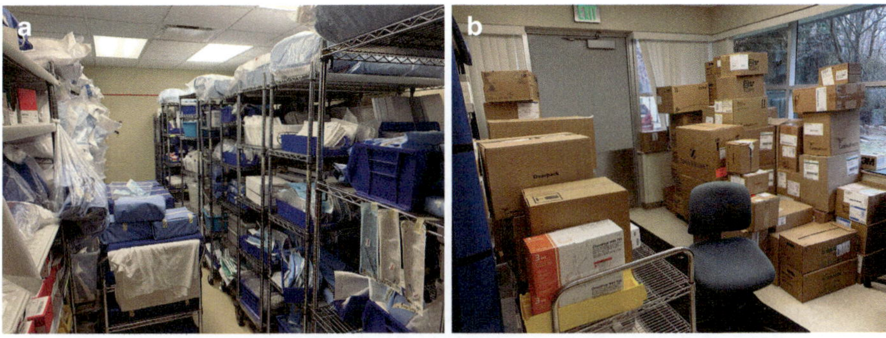

Fig. 10.4 Ambulatory surgery center storage (**a**) Sterile storage (**b**) Disposable storage

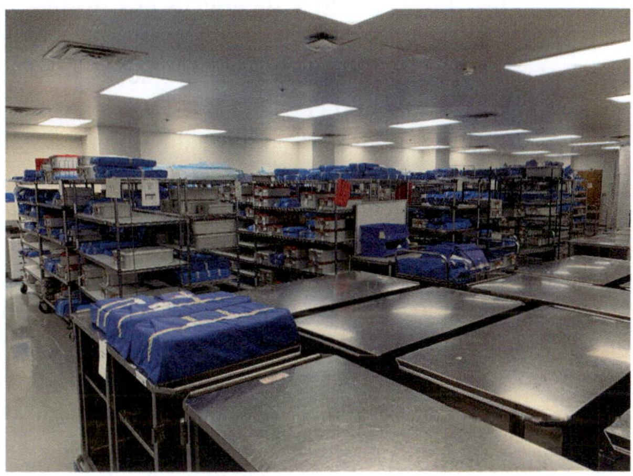

Fig. 10.5 Hospital storage. While space dedicated to instrument and equipment storage will vary significantly between hospitals, this represents an example of three separate rooms utilized for storage in one hospital system

the best of which can be debated, but may be as follows: (1) primary repair with hinged knee brace [1], (2) primary repair with internal augmentation [2], (3) conversion to more constrained implants [4–7], and (4) a combination of each option. Any of these options requires more than just routine implants, instrumentation, and supplies. It may sound strange for those of us working in the hospital environment, but even heavier braided suture may not be routinely stocked unless you have requested it. Depending on your preference, you would need to have certain types of suture, perhaps certain suture anchors, hinged knee braces (which may or may not be readily stocked), and of course more constrained implant options. The latter poses an even larger challenge given limitations in space and sterile processing as well as advanced vendor negotiations. This example typifies the need for a thorough preoperative plan, so that ultimately you choose the right patients and can therefore rely less on rare special equipment needs.

Instruments

Most surgeons are used to walking into the OR and having the instruments ready. They may or may not know how many trays are even required to do their cases, but for the majority of total joint replacements, that number is not insignificant. In a large hospital, there is typically ample storage for such equipment. In an ASC, that is not necessarily the case. The way that different facilities manage instruments and implants varies based on space and general operating procedures. Some facilities will have instruments they purchased or are on consignment. Others will require vendors to bring instruments in or coordinate with affiliated hospital systems to stock appropriate instruments as needed. Limited space often means making arrangements for some devices and vendor trays "just in time." Hospitals often have storage racks allocated for loaner instruments, whereas most ASCs do not have space for this. Instead, ASCs default to just-in-time delivery arrangements often 24 h prior to surgery for specific implants. Again, these deliveries are scheduled and the contents pre-determined to meet the needs of the case. Patient selection and preparation dictate this process and if the work has not been done on the front end, the options will be limited if additional equipment is ultimately required as mentioned above.

The way that surgeons and staff utilize instruments will also vary. For example, when the surgeon has completed a portion of the case and certain instruments are no longer needed, they are handed off for processing. This routinely happens throughout the case in an ASC, and not just at the end. Other strategies can be employed to improve instrument efficiency such as the development of a "mini-bar" for when instruments are missing or dropped or contaminated. With this strategy, entire trays are not opened for a single instrument, rather single instruments are packed individually. Having individual instruments peel-packed and available in a set location ("mini-bar") allows for redundancy when needed without significant cost and logistics of full sets.

Managing instrument utilization efficiently can also be approached proactively by critically assessing the instrumentation trays being used. Most surgeons use the same instruments for their cases. Yet, in most hospitals those instruments come from a variety of different instrument sets. It would not be uncommon in a hospital to open an osteotome set that contains 12 different straight and curved osteotomes even though you may only use a 1/2 inch curved osteotome for your case. Similarly, most hospitals have an "ortho basic" set with a mix of dozens of instruments that are commonly used in any orthopedic procedure. At our hospital, we have looked at this extensively and began creating dedicated hip and knee instrument sets. This process brought the number of instrument trays down from 9 full trays down to 1 small tray for total hips and 1 small tray for partial and total knees (Fig. 10.6a, b). In addition, working with your vendors to decrease the number of instruments needed to be more efficient can substantially reduce the implant-specific instrumentation needed (Fig. 10.6c, d). This equates to not just fewer trays, but faster turnover, improved efficiency intraoperatively, easier cross-training of staff, less space requirements, faster sterile processing, and instrument replacement. All of this decreases time and

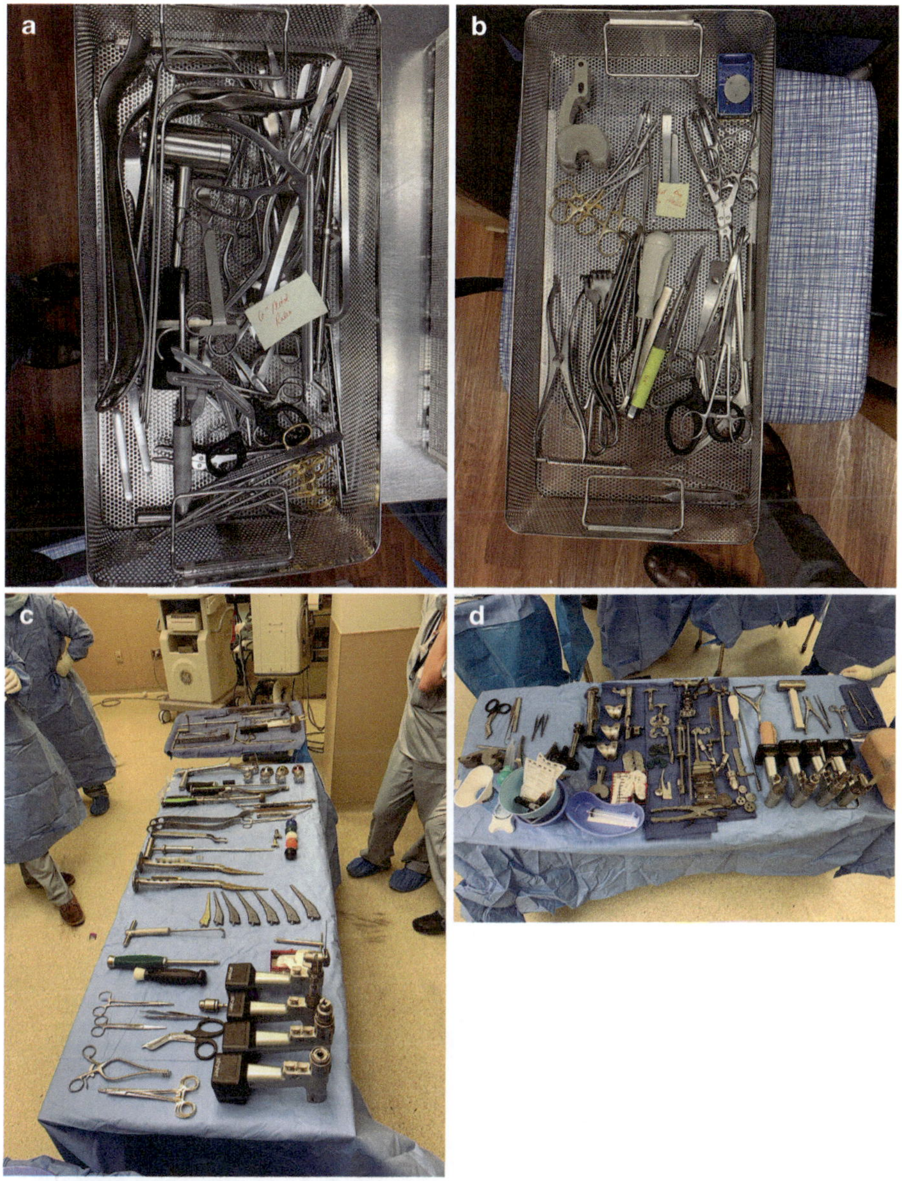

Fig. 10.6 Instrumentation for (**a**) total hip arthroplasty and (**b**) total knee arthroplasty. Complete operating room instrumentation including implant instrumentation for (**c**) total hip arthroplasty and (**d**) total knee arthroplasty

cost associated with each case. Cichos et al. recently reported on the value of optimizing surgical instrumentation and demonstrated that after implementing lean principles they were able to reduce instrumentation by 55% for a total annual cost savings of $270,976 [8].

Sterile Processing

Due to more consolidated and few overall sets, there must be an efficient process for turning over instruments. Some of these have been mentioned above, but a more comprehensive understanding of sterile processing and instrument management can clearly demonstrate the challenges ASCs face. Leadership must have a defined and well-communicated plan as to how to execute instrument turnover, including when sets will be needed again and for which patient/OR. The decontamination department is much more consolidated in an ASC compared to a hospital (Figs. 10.7 and 10.8). First, there are no cart washers in most ASCs, meaning carts require manual cleaning before reuse. Dirty instruments go on the same countertop for cleaning as the instruments that were "barely used" creating tighter working conditions for the staff on the sterilization side of the process. This is in contrast to most hospital sterilization departments that have separate areas for contaminated versus clean but used instruments. Planning and facility design are critical to the success of these processes at the ASC. With limited counter space, sink, and general cleaning space, instruments must move into the washers and through the pass-thru window quickly

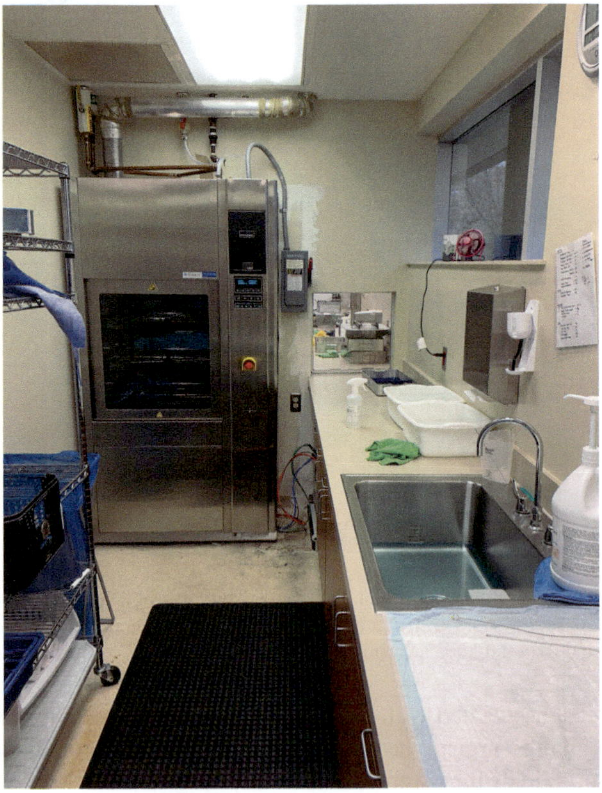

Fig. 10.7 Ambulatory surgery center sterile processing. These images represent the sterile processing space for a four-room ambulatory facility

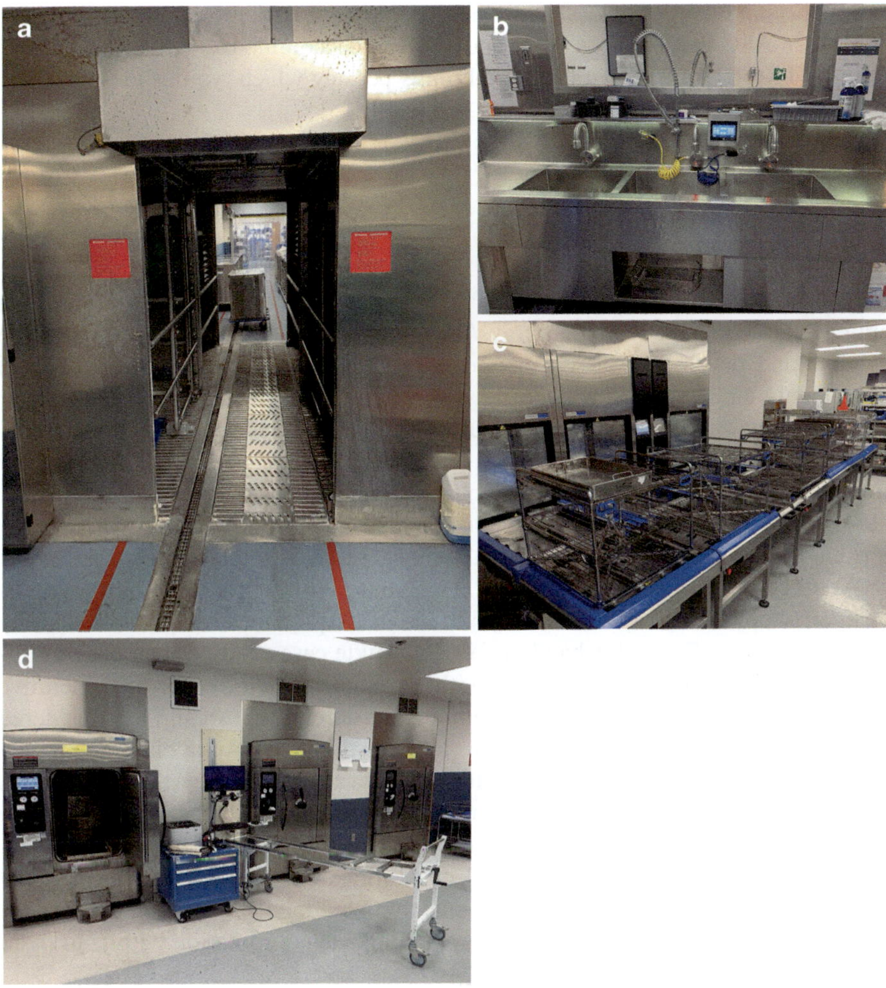

Fig. 10.8 Hospital sterile processing. There are several stages to sterile processing in hospitals and a significant amount of space and equipment is dedicated to processing. (**a**) Instrument cart cleaner. (**b**) Soak and sonic sinks. (**c**) Instrument washers on conveyer belt. (**d**) Steris sterilizers

to make space for incoming dirty instruments entering decontamination. It is also imperative that certain trays are identified and prioritized if they are needed again on the same day.

If you ask most surgeons about sterile processing, it is likely they have never even seen the facility or equipment at their hospital. Figures 10.7 and 10.8 demonstrate the clear contrast between ASC and hospital decontamination and sterilization areas. While it is possible in some larger hospitals to perform high-volume joint replacement, depending on the size of the ASC it is fascinating to think that in that small space they can process similar volumes of total joint instrumentation as the larger hospital facilities in less time. The sterilization area demonstrated in Fig. 10.7 is from an ASC that between 0700 and 1700 can accommodate two surgeons performing 10 total joints. That is 20 total joints per day which typifies the efficiency despite lack of space.

An ASC is an Island

At an ASC, you have what you have. Preparation is critical. What are your bail-out options? Do you have redundant trays/instruments? Diligent coordination with the vendors and developing an understanding of what the options are for different instruments and implants will be necessary. The ASC management needs clear arrangements with the vendors for ensuring options are available and pricing is pre-negotiated. For example, if you are in a situation where there is an intraoperative fracture or soft tissue compromise, you may want to have cerclage cables, basic plates, and screws or perhaps more constrained implants available. If you are performing a partial knee replacement you will want to have a total knee available.

Another consideration is imaging. Does your facility have digital radiographs or fluoroscopy available? For total joints, is that equipment adequate? A facility may have a mini C-arm for hand or foot and ankle cases, but do they have a full-size C-arm or portable radiographs with a sufficient plate to get intraoperative imaging when needed? Other less commonly used items that should be considered are different suture options and perhaps anchors if needed. Appreciating you may not have access to your office or hospital PACS system from the ASC OR requires either printing images in advance or bringing a device that can access those images. Operating rooms, in general, may not vary greatly in size between ASCs and hospitals, but the equipment and capabilities in the ORs can be different (Fig. 10.9). Knowing what you need is one thing but knowing what you may need and making sure it is available requires planning and coordination with your management team.

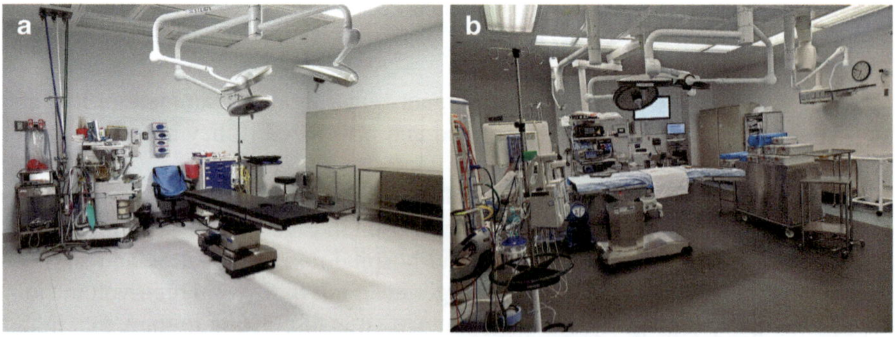

Fig. 10.9 (**a**) Ambulatory surgery center operating room and (**b**) Hospital Operating Room

Durable medical equipment (DME) represents another topic. Although less commonly used in joint replacement, every facility has different policies when it comes to stocking DME. Smaller facilities may actually bring braces in for specific procedures while others stock a variety of common DME products. There are multiple different DME vendors and working with your management team to ensure you have products that are sufficient to cover your needs is important. In some cases, if you have DME available in your office, a reasonable solution is to provide it prior to surgery and have the patient bring it with them. Alternatively, you can provide your prescriptions for DME in advance and they can be procured independently and brought in. The last thing you want is for the surgery to go well and the patient is unable to leave when they are cleared because a walker is not available.

Medications are often determined by the ASC drug formulary. This formulary is typically decided and voted on at the medical executive committee and/or board meetings. Having a formal process often keeps the formulary consolidated to a list of options that all surgeons will use. This is different from hospitals that have a breadth of options and the capacity to cater to each individual surgeon. That may limit options as far as antibiotics, local anesthetics, or additional custom protocols surgeons prefer. As a general rule, if it is not on the formulary, unless you ask for it, it will not be there.

Everything Moves Faster

Your surgical technique may be the same, but everything else moves faster in an ASC. Even though staffing levels are typically less than at most hospitals, the staff is uniquely selected based on expertise and efficiency to accommodate the appropriate volume required. The surgeon has less variability in staff and the staff knows what to expect when showing up for those surgery days. In most circumstances, ASC staff have specialized training in the procedures being performed and if surgeons operate regularly at the ASC, they have those preferences down to a tee. Staff call-ins are more difficult to manage logistically but are much less common in a well-run ASC and contingency plans are quickly mobilized when necessary. In general, because the ASC is a smaller environment the culture of the organization evokes a strong sense of responsibility and ownership at the staff level. In the event of call-ins, it is often the ASC leadership that will fill in the gaps due to lean staffing models and those leaders are cross-trained to do so efficiently.

In many cases, surgeons will bring their own staff, whether it be a physician assistant (PA) or nurse practitioner (NP), a private scrub tech or first assistant (FA), or even a registered nurse (RN). For those who do not bring additional staff, the ASC will provide appropriate staffing. In either scenario, there is a culture of efficiency and productivity. Understanding this culture is drastically different than a typical hospital staffing structure. Expectations of ASC staff are much higher. First assistants and/or PAs in ASCs are expected not only to assist in positioning and in surgery, but the entire staff, regardless of their position, helps with setup and cleanup. The same thing applies to the nurses and the techs. Again, the staffing ratios are less in the ASC environment and there are often no environmental services departments to clean the operating rooms between cases. Even though the number of staff is fewer, turnover remains much faster as clinical staff rise to the occasion and work harder to facilitate smooth transitions between the cases.

For many surgeons entering an ASC for the first time, this can be an adjustment. It is not uncommon in many hospitals to have an hour or more turnover time between cases. Most ASCs have turnovers closer to 10–15 min. When considering that time, surgeons often have to adapt and make changes to their workflow in order to maintain the schedule. There are no shift changes like we see at the hospital and many ASCs provide lunch for the staff and surgeons so that the downtime can be as productive as possible and efficiencies maximized.

Anesthesia

Perhaps one of the most important advances in joint replacement surgery is a comprehensive understanding of managing pain. There is an entire chapter in this book dedicated to anesthesia, but in an ASC the importance of efficient anesthesia protocols cannot be understated. To accommodate a fast recovery, short-acting local anesthetic agents and minimal narcotic use are preferred. However, they place constraints on the surgeon, requiring a more coordinated approach for prepping, draping, and performing the surgery. Thus, the surgeon has to carefully choose the cases that can be performed in the ASC due to time limitations from the short-acting anesthesia.

Our preference has been a single-shot spinal for outpatient anesthesia using a short-acting agent such as lidocaine or low-dose hyperbaric bupiviaine [9]. Working with the anesthesiologist at your ASC to adjust dosing based on your surgical techniques, timing and protocols is critical and may take time. Unlike the hospital environment where patients with prolonged blocks can easily be admitted and monitored, in an ASC the impact is longer recovery room time which is detrimental to the entire ASC process. Longer recovery time results in a longer wait time for families, decreasing waiting room capacity, increased staff required for that patient, decreasing availability for other patients or cross-utilization in other areas, and overall increased marginal cost of the case. As in many aspects of the ASC, a failure or delay in one area affects the entire process adversely.

Concurrent with the shift toward neuraxial anesthesia has been an expansion of multimodal pain pathways. Medications are determined by the ASC drug formulary, so if you use specific agents or multimodal pathways, or have certain preferences for nerve blocks, you will need to ensure the facility approves and stocks those for your cases in advance.

Physical Therapy

Typically, most ASCs do not have physical therapy on site. There remains some debate on whether or not having a physical therapist in the recovery room provides tangible patient benefit. That said, surgeons have different preferences for postoperative therapy and options are available. Many ASCs actually provide the nursing staff training on postoperative recovery protocols and the staff is cross-trained to fill that need. These requirements may vary based on individual discharge criteria, but a protocol is recommended to ensure quality, safety, and reproducible processes in the center.

In some cases, it is possible to bring therapists from your own office. Certain facilities contract with outside companies to provide therapy services directly at the ASC. There can be some advantages to contracted arrangements from an economic standpoint. Having an outside therapy company on site alleviates the burden on your staff, which therefore decreases staffing needs and can effectively increase throughput. These arrangements may or may not require direct compensation from the ASC but more often than not the therapy company provides those services independently and manages any additional billing directly. Alternatively, some therapy companies will provide these services without cost, in hopes that they will develop a relationship with the patient to provide home or outpatient therapy in the postoperative period.

For example, following surgery at the ASC, the therapy company does an initial visit to the patient in the recovery room by a licensed therapist. The patient is treated with manual passive range of motion education and evaluation. They provide a basic introduction to bed exercises (i.e., quad sets, heel slides, straight leg raise, etc.). The patient will be educated on using an assist device, fitted for that device and ambulate a certain distance (i.e., 200–300 feet). Safety and stability while using stairs will be reviewed. Of note, your facility may or may not have stairs available and if you are just starting a joint replacement program either the facility or the therapy group will have to procure appropriate stairs. Once this is complete, the patient is discharged home.

References

1. Bohl DD, Wetters NG, Del Gaizo DJ, Jacobs JJ, Rosenberg AG, Della Valle CJ. Repair of intraoperative injury to the medial collateral ligament during primary Total knee arthroplasty. J Bone Joint Surg Am. 2016;98(1):35–9.
2. Shahi A, Tan TL, Tarabichi S, Maher A, Della Valle C, Saleh UH. Primary repair of iatrogenic medial collateral ligament injury during TKA: a modified technique. J Arthroplast. 2015;30(5):854–7.
3. Leopold SS, McStay C, Klafeta K, Jacobs JJ, Berger RA, Rosenberg AG. Primary repair of intraoperative disruption of the medical collateral ligament during total knee arthroplasty. J Bone Joint Surg Am. 2001;83-a(1):86–91.

4. Lee GC, Lotke PA. Management of intraoperative medial collateral ligament injury during TKA. Clin Orthop Relat Res. 2011;469(1):64–8.
5. Hartford JM, Goodman SB, Schurman DJ, Knoblick G. Complex primary and revision total knee arthroplasty using the condylar constrained prosthesis: an average 5-year follow-up. J Arthroplast. 1998;13(4):380–7.
6. Callaghan JJ, O'Rourke MR, Liu SS. The role of implant constraint in revision total knee arthroplasty: not too little, not too much. J Arthroplast. 2005;20(4 Suppl 2):41–3.
7. Rosenberg AG, Verner JJ, Galante JO. Clinical results of total knee revision using the total condylar III prosthesis. Clin Orthop Relat Res. 1991;273:83–90.
8. Cichos KH, Hyde ZB, Mabry SE, Ghanem ES, Brabston EW, Hayes LW, et al. Optimization of orthopedic surgical instrument trays: lean principles to reduce fixed operating room expenses. J Arthroplast. 2019;34(12):2834–40.
9. Frisch NB, Darrith B, Hansen DC, Wells A, Sanders S, Berger RA. Single-dose lidocaine spinal anesthesia in hip and knee arthroplasty. Arthroplast today. 2018;4(2):236–9.

Chapter 11
Same-Day Discharge in the Hospital: Resources and Program Elements

Gregory G. Polkowski and Michael D. Gabbard

Introduction

Modern advancements in total joint arthroplasty (TJA) techniques promoting rapid recovery, including immediate weight bearing, multimodal pain regimens, spinal anesthesia, and blood management strategies have culminated in the rise of outpatient TJA [1–6]. The initial transition to same-day TJA occurred in the ambulatory surgery center (ASC) setting. In this environment, the surgeon maintained complete control of the patient experience, and it allowed the process to be refined, demonstrated adequate safety, and led to the establishment of patient selection criteria that makes same-day TJA feasible. Surgeons view this as an opportunity to improve efficiency and minimize potential complications of prolonged time spent in the hospital, which in turn results in improved patient satisfaction with their joint replacement experience [7]. While there may be fewer obstacles to the implementation of outpatient TJA in an ASC, there are numerous compelling reasons to consider it in a hospital setting.

Reasons to Consider Outpatient TJA in Hospital Setting

Compared to ASCs, many large hospitals are characterized by having cumbersome and frequently archaic processes that are difficult to control and change. The bureaucratic quagmire creates frustration for both surgeons and patients. However, performing outpatient TJA in a large hospital setting can still be attractive for several

G. G. Polkowski (✉) · M. D. Gabbard
Department of Orthopaedic Surgery, Vanderbilt University Medical Center, Nashville, TN, USA
e-mail: gregory.polkowski@vumc.org

R. M. Meneghini, L. T. Buller (eds.), *Outpatient Hip and Knee Replacement*,
https://doi.org/10.1007/978-3-031-27037-6_11

reasons. The most compelling reason is to provide a better overall patient experience and improve patient satisfaction. In general, the time a patient spends in the hospital is not enjoyable. The transition from admission to surgery to recovery, and, finally, discharge is fragmented and inefficient.

Large hospitals have conflicting interests including high volumes of patients, hourly employees, numerous trainees in multiple fields, and lack of incentives for timely completion of tasks. These issues can lead to significant compromises in efficiency. Patients often experience large delays at multiple levels including in the post-anesthesia care unit (PACU) and waiting on inpatient bed assignments. These delays can often result in missed physical therapy on the day of surgery, delayed meeting with case managers, and ultimately result in significantly increased time before readiness for discharge. This can be a source of frustration to patients and their families, resulting in dissatisfaction with their experience. A well-designed outpatient TJA program would offer the opportunity to mitigate this.

The following example, while not always typical, demonstrates the challenges of delivering care at our 1000+ bed tertiary-referral academic medical center. A patient may wait over an hour in a crowded waiting room, and spend another 1–2 h in the holding room while a new nurse struggles to achieve intravenous access. They are interviewed by a medical student, anesthesia resident, and eventually anesthesia attending on three separate occasions. The surgical case cart could not be found during the room turnover, delaying the start time another 30 min. Once in the operating room, the anesthesia trainee struggles to administer spinal anesthesia, and eventually the operation is performed. The hospital is relatively full, and there is a "PACU delay" of another 20 min while the patient begins their recovery in the operating room. Because of the hospital capacity issues, instead of going to the orthopedic floor 60–90 min after they come out of surgery, the patient spends 4–5 h in the recovery room. They wait another hour for the designated patient transportation personnel to take them to their room, and by the time they arrive, they have missed the dinner food service, and the physical therapy team has gone home for the day. They are awakened every couple of hours at night for nursing assessments, vital signs, and phlebotomy. Before the sun comes up, they are visited by a medical student, an orthopaedic resident, and eventually the attending surgeon. Even if they are doing well, there is another delay before they have their first inpatient physical therapy session and finally start to walk. Because of hospital policy, the case managers and discharge planners, who are obligated to process every patient, eventually see the patient and perform their assessment, even though the patient does not require home health services, and already has an outpatient physical therapy appointment arranged for the day after their discharge. Once deemed appropriate for discharge to home, the nursing discharge process can take another 1–2 h, depending upon patient load, and transportation via wheelchair to their car may require another 45 min. Not all of these delays occur for every patient, but the level of frustration that is felt as they do add up can be maddening. To optimize patient satisfaction, then, it stands to reason that minimizing the number of steps the patient is required to experience, in the large hospital setting, will reduce the number of delays and improve overall satisfaction.

Patient safety is another reason to consider outpatient TJA, even in the hospital setting. In 2014, the CDC reported that medical errors were the third leading cause of death, behind heart disease and cancer [8]. Each step in the patient-care pathway during a hospitalization, regardless of the need for hospitalization, creates an opportunity for error. The longer the time and the more steps the patient is exposed to, the greater the chance of a medical error occurring. Even though a tremendous amount of effort has been put forth to reduce hospital error, the simplest way to avoid it is not to spend time in the hospital.

Another appealing reason to consider outpatient TJA in the hospital setting is to maintain your individual value as a surgeon to the hospital system. Formerly, total hip (THA) and knee arthroplasty (TKA) were considered inpatient-only procedures, which provided inherent value to the total joint replacement surgeon performing these procedures in the hospital setting. However, as TKA and THA are removed from the Centers for Medicare and Medicaid Services Inpatient-Only list, it has resulted in an overall paradigm change. In the absence of the hospital diagnosis-related group (DRG) associated with inpatient admission designation, the value created by reducing the length of stay from 1 to2 days to zero days by proactively launching an outpatient surgery program aligns the incentives of the hospital administrators (length of stay) with the surgeon and patients (patient experience), creating value. With coordinated efforts between surgeons and hospital administration, an outpatient TJA program can result in mutual success.

Implementation of Outpatient TJA in Hospital Setting

Implementation of an outpatient TJA in a hospital setting requires considerable planning, which begins with the evaluation of potential barriers to success. This can be accomplished by first mapping the process from arrival at the hospital through discharge. It is important to identify each segment of the patient-care pathway, the key players involved in each step, and what the limitations are to progress to the subsequent step. Common obstacles identified can include an excess number of people involved in the process, shift worker mentality of individuals, and an overall large number of steps required to meet discharge criteria. It is important to critically evaluate each individual item and determine whether it is optimal to relocate it in the process, enhance its effectiveness, or eliminate it completely. Oftentimes the most effective choices are aimed at simplifying the process. Relocating steps that can be performed prior to surgery and eliminating all unnecessary steps on the date of surgery will maximize efficiency and the likelihood of a successful outpatient TJA. For example, one path to same-day discharge may involve the patient moving from the PACU to the orthopedic floor to undergo physical therapy, and then eventual discharge. A more efficient process, though, is to make the transition from the hospital room discharge model to a PACU discharge model, in which the patient is immediately assessed in the recovery room. This involves removal of numerous patient transport steps, delays in PT, involvement of case manager/social worker, and delays in discharge medications and orders. This ultimately results in a substantially more efficient process.

Another aspect of implementing a successful outpatient TJA program in the hospital setting requires organizing a multidisciplinary team and achieving buy-in towards the common goal of outpatient TJA. Delivering the same consistent message to each person at every step of the patient-care path is essential, and more difficult in the hospital setting compared with the ASC. Our experience has shown that this process is best achieved when this is a surgeon-led effort. In order to transform a multidisciplinary group of individuals, with previously misaligned priorities, into a cooperative effort requires significant engagement. Overcoming the potential energy to get the proverbial ball rolling can be a challenge. One helpful process is to create a "program" or "trial" at the hospital and give it a name, so it is recognizable. When beginning this process at our institution, we named it *H.E.R.O., (High Efficiency Reconstructive Orthopaedics),* which allowed those involved in the care of HERO patients to feel like they were part of a patient-care process that was different than the typical hospital experience.

The importance of the "Team" in the success of an outpatient TJA program in the hospital setting cannot be overstated. Being part of a special process can generate excitement among team members. It is also important to emphasize teamwork and accentuate the importance of each individual's role in achieving success. After-hours activities or sponsored lunches can be tools used to enhance group bonding and reinforce the importance of their roles. Large groups need a big push to make changes, but if individuals feel they are a part of something larger than themselves it can be a significant motivating factor. Following the implementation of a program, continue to elicit feedback from all members of the team and consider changes based on this feedback. There will be many opportunities for continued improvement.

Other considerations for an outpatient TJA program in the hospital setting include patient selection criteria. There are various methods and recommendations for this, but ultimately the selection of appropriate patients that can be successful in your program will lead to the best results. It is important to not try to make outpatient TJA fit for those who are uncomfortable with the idea or who have medical comorbidities requiring full hospitalization for management and monitoring. Despite the increasing frequency of outpatient TJA, a recent study by Meneghini et al. reported only 54.5% of patients were aware that outpatient TJA was even an option and 54% expected to spend two or more nights in the hospital [9]. This demonstrates that among patients who will be candidates for outpatient TJA, preoperative education surrounding expectations is extremely important to alleviate anxiety and prepare patients and their caregivers. In general, it is preferable to schedule potential outpatient cases earlier in the day to allow ample time to reach necessary discharge criteria. Coordinating with physical therapists and making them aware of potential outpatient candidates in advance will allow for prioritization and the earliest feasible PT for these patients. It is important to keep in mind that even when outpatient joint replacement is the primary plan, it is not always successful for various reasons. However, an attractive benefit of an outpatient TJA program in a hospital setting versus an ASC is that when a patient fails discharge, it is typically a seamless transition back to the traditional inpatient model.

Experiences with Outpatient TJA in Hospital Setting in the Literature

The majority of peer-reviewed literature on outpatient TJA involves patients who receive their care in the ASC setting, and the data on outpatient surgery in the hospital setting is fairly limited. There are a few reports of implementation of outpatient TJA in hospital settings in the literature. First, Gogineni et al. report on the transition to outpatient hip and knee arthroplasty at a large, academic hospital [10]. All of their TJA procedures were performed as per their standard protocols with the only difference for the outpatient group being that they received PT in the PACU and were discharged home the same day if criteria were met. Seventy-nine percent (83/105) of patients were successfully discharged home the same day. Predictors of same-day discharge included TKA, shorter duration of surgery, and longer first ambulation distance in PACU. Average time in PACU prior to ambulation was 186 min and average overall PACU stay prior to discharge was 351 min. The most common causes for failed same-day discharge were orthostatic hypotension, patient decision, urinary retention, and nausea. There were only two emergency department visits within 48 h of surgery, one for syncope and one for traumatic wound dehiscence. This study demonstrates the successful implementation of outpatient TJA in a large, multispecialty, tertiary care hospital.

A prospective study at a public, university-affiliated hospital in Chile reported on their experience with a novel outpatient THA program [11]. In a carefully selected group of patients, 68/72 (94.4%) were successfully discharged home the same day. Patients spent an average of 5 h in the recovery room prior to discharge. Three patients required overnight stays in the recovery room (two for nausea, one for transportation issues), and only one required transition to inpatient status due to prolonged anesthesia effects. There were no emergency department visits during the first week after surgery. All patients reported they were satisfied with their outpatient track choice and would recommend it to others. This study provides another example of implementation of outpatient joint replacement in a hospital setting with a high rate of success and patient satisfaction and few complications.

Schultz et al. report on the implementation of an accelerated recovery and outpatient TJA program at a County hospital [12]. They describe their experience in creating a multidisciplinary team aimed at maximizing efficiency in TJA. They compared 108 TJA patients after implementation of their protocol to the 108 immediately prior. They report a decrease in length of stay (3.4 days to 1.6), decrease in overall complication rate (21% to 7%), increase in discharge to home (72% to 92%), and decreased overall mean total cost of TJA by approximately 25%. Despite identifying a lack of strong social support systems as a unique challenge, they demonstrated success with an accelerated recovery program even in a large, county hospital.

Conclusion

Outpatient TJA continues to gain momentum and will be performed with increasing frequency in the future. While implementing an outpatient TJA program in a large hospital setting has some distinct challenges in comparison to an ASC, there remains good reason to consider it. Outpatient TJA provides an opportunity to improve patient experience and offers value to the hospital system. The most pertinent criteria for successful implementation remain proper patient selection and education. Efforts in preparation, coordination, and education prior to the day of surgery allow outpatient TJA to be feasible. For the in-hospital experience, cutting down the size of the process and developing an engaged, multidisciplinary team is critical to the process. Continually eliciting feedback from these team members and making applicable changes will ensure reproducible success. Lastly, there will be patients who fail to meet discharge criteria for various reasons, and an attractive benefit of an outpatient TJA program in a hospital setting is the option of a seamless transition back to the traditional inpatient model when deemed necessary.

References

1. Sculco PK, Pagnano MW. Perioperative solutions for rapid recovery joint arthroplasty: get ahead and stay ahead. J Arthroplast. 2015;30(4):518–20.
2. Hozack WJ, Matsen-Ko L. Rapid recovery after hip and knee arthroplasty: a process and a destination. J Arthroplast. 2015;30(4):517.
3. Berend KR, Lombardi AV, Mallory TH. Rapid recovery protocol for peri-operative care of total hip and total knee arthroplasty patients. Surg Technol Int. 2004;13:239.
4. Russo MW, Parks NL, Hamilton WG. Perioperative pain management and anesthesia: a critical component to rapid recovery Total joint arthroplasty. Orthop Clin North Am. 2017;48(4):401–5.
5. Galbraith AS, McGloughlin E, Cashman J. Enhanced recovery protocols in total joint arthroplasty: a review of the literature and their implementation. Ir J Med Sci. 2018;187(1):97–109.
6. Hoffmann JD, Kusnezov NA, Dunn JC, Zarkadis NJ, Goodman GP, Berger RA. The shift to same-day outpatient joint arthroplasty: a systematic review. J Arthroplast. 2018;33(4):1265–74.
7. Hamilton DF, Lane JV, Gaston P, Patton JT, Macdonald D, Simpson AH, Howie CR. What determines patient satisfaction with surgery? A prospective cohort study of 4709 patients following total joint replacement. BMJ Open. 2013;3(4):e002525.
8. Makary MA, Daniel M. Medical error—the third leading cause of death in the US. BMJ. 2016;3:353.
9. Meneghini RM, Ziemba-Davis M. Patient perceptions regarding outpatient hip and knee arthroplasties. J Arthroplast. 2017;32(9):2701–5.
10. Gogineni HC, Gray CF, Prieto HA, Deen JT, Boezaart AP, Parvataneni HK. Transition to outpatient total hip and knee arthroplasty: experience at an academic tertiary care center. Arthroplast Today. 2019;5(1):100–5.

11. Paredes O, Ñuñez R, Klaber I. Successful initial experience with a novel outpatient total hip arthroplasty program in a public health system in Chile. Int Orthop. 2018;42(8):1783–7.
12. Schultz BJ, Segovia N, Castillo TN. Successful implementation of an accelerated recovery and outpatient total joint arthroplasty program at a county hospital. J Am Acad Orthop Surg Glob Res Rev. 2019;3(9):e110.

Chapter 12
Discharge the Day of Surgery: Strategies to Optimize and Discharge Criteria

Joshua C. Rozell, Dimitri E. Delagrammaticas, and Raymond H. Kim

Preoperative Visit

Expectations should be discussed with the patient during the first visit when surgery is scheduled. This involves clearly identifying appropriate candidates based on medical, technical, and social factors, setting a tone of expectation for outpatient recovery, and delivering a consistent and coordinated message from the surgeon, mid-level providers, scheduler, and operating room facility. The decision to enroll a patient in a same-day discharge program should be shared. The patient should understand that recovery at home is very different from recovery in a hospital setting. There are certain advantages to in-home recoveries, such as recovery in familiar surroundings, better sleep quality, less noise, less exposure to potential infections, and having a support system of family and friends [1, 2]. The preoperative visit also involves a thorough discussion of medications including their purpose and intended schedule of use, scheduling and explaining the role and frequency of outpatient physical therapy, and setting up postoperative visits. As some patients may have difficulty retaining all of the details of the presurgical conversation, including key caregivers and family members in the visit as well as giving patients a written total joint replacement recovery guide to take home and read is helpful to reinforce the key aspects of the preoperative visit. Moreover, since the patient goes home on the same day, the work typically performed by a social worker in the hospital setting

J. C. Rozell
NYU Langone Health, New York, NY, USA
e-mail: Joshua.rozell@nyulangone.org

D. E. Delagrammaticas
Central Coast Orthopedic Group, San Luis Obispo, CA, USA

R. H. Kim (✉)
The Steadman Clinic, Vail, CO, USA
e-mail: rkim@thesteadmanclinic.com

R. M. Meneghini, L. T. Buller (eds.), *Outpatient Hip and Knee Replacement*,
https://doi.org/10.1007/978-3-031-27037-6_12

falls on the surgical team, much of which should be coordinated well before the surgical date. Coordinating each step of the postoperative disposition before the surgical date ensures that the recovery proceeds seamlessly without any delays or miscommunication in receiving the appropriate care. Many practices offer a preoperative joint replacement class [3]. These group sessions are often led by a nurse or nurse practitioner who reviews the surgical process from start to finish with the patients. This also serves as a forum for patients to ask questions and voice any concerns. Having multiple avenues to deliver the preoperative message ensures that patients can, depending on learning styles, take advantage of classes, lectures, videos, pictures, and information packets to be knowledgeable and well-equipped to succeed with the same-day discharge on the day of surgery [4].

Patient Selection

Not all patients are appropriate candidates for same-day discharge. An important aspect of performing an early discharge or outpatient arthroplasty is appropriately selecting patients to avoid putting them at undue risk either in the ambulatory setting or at home. To this end, evaluation for inclusion involves an assessment of a patient's medical comorbidities, social and living situation, psychological preparedness, and motivation. It is important to have a consistent tool by which patients can predictably be chosen for discharge on the same day or within 23 h. The Outpatient Arthroplasty Risk Assessment (OARA) score is one such tool validated to identify patients who may or may not be candidates for same-day discharge [5, 6]. The OARA score assigns a point value to questions pertaining to medical conditions in specific body systems and a summation score that can be interpreted to identify patients appropriate for outpatient surgery. Working with a consistent perioperative internal medicine practitioner who understands the key program characteristics, such as recovery protocols, anesthetic techniques, surgeon experience, optimized care pathways, and is involved in a routine multidisciplinary care conference is a critical aspect of identifying and optimizing patients for outpatient arthroplasty. Understandably, the availability of a perioperative internal medicine specialist dedicated solely to TJA patients may not be available in many practice settings; however, the concept should serve as a model for consistent and outpatient-focused preoperative medical evaluations [5].

Anesthesia and Pain Management

On the day of surgery the entire patient experience should be as streamlined as possible. Over the last several years, anesthesia pain protocols have made significant advancements, allowing surgery to be performed under a short-acting spinal anesthetic with a multimodal pain approach, utilizing minimal to no opioids. The approach to pain management should involve taking a patient's pain history, preoperative narcotic exposure, and an evaluation of their overall response to pain. Involvement, coordination, and buy-in between both the surgeon and anesthesiologist in developing a rapid recovery total joint protocol are imperative to maintain consistency, efficiency, and safety [7]. Patient, as well as facility-related factors, may affect the exact details of the protocol, but in general avoiding inhaled anesthetics in favor of regional anesthesia and intravenous sedation is preferable to minimize nausea, dizziness, and excessive sedation. These side effects of general anesthesia may contribute to potential failed progression through the postoperative discharge criteria. Furthermore, avoiding longer than necessary spinal, as well as utilizing local or regional local anesthetic infiltration that avoids motor blockade can mitigate the risk of urinary retention and delayed mobilization [8].

Below is an example anesthesia regimen for the surgical episode, beginning in the holding area and finishing in the recovery area. In general, most protocols will involve a preoperative pain medication cocktail consisting of non-narcotic medications to supplement the postoperative pain regimen. For knee replacement, regional anesthetic infiltration in the form of an adductor canal block can provide partial blockage of pain in the knee and avoid motor involvement. Data regarding the use of adductor canal blocks for total knee arthroplasty is mixed, with some studies advocating for blocks while others report sufficient analgesia with periarticular injection alone [9–11]. Adductor canal blocks typically fail to completely anesthetize the lateral and posterior aspect of the knee, so supplemental local infiltration may be required [12]. To improve the efficiency of the operative day, the spinal and/or block should ideally be performed outside of the operating room, either in the holding area or an induction room.

Preoperatively:

- Acetaminophen 1000 mg PO.
- Pregabalin 150 mg PO; Dose can be decreased to 75 mg for elderly patients.
- Celecoxib 400 mg PO; Dose can be decreased to 200 mg for elderly patients.
- For TKA Only: Adductor Canal Nerve Block: Ropivacaine 0.2%, 20 mL.
- Midazolam 2 mg IV for sedation during the block/spinal.

Spinal (Titrated to surgeon speed or case complexity) placed preoperatively before patient arrives in the operating room:

- Mepivacaine 1.5% Isobaric 45 mg (3 mL). Should last 2–3 h.
- Mepivacaine 1.5% Isobaric 60 mg (4 mL) for slower surgeons or revisions.
- Bupivacaine 0.75% Hyperbaric 12–15 mg for very slow surgeons. This will delay the discharge of patients from PACU due to prolong motor blockade.

Intraoperatively

- Propofol Infusion: Dose from 50–100 μg/kg/min.
- Decadron 0.15 mg/kg with a maximum dose of 15 mg.
- Ketamine 0.5 mg/kg up to 50 mg; Decrease dose for elderly patients.
- Ketorolac 30 mg IV; May need to hold in patients with renal insufficiency.
- Ondansetron 4 mg IV.

Recovery Room

- Fentanyl 25 μg IV to maximum dose of 100 μg available as needed until the patient can safely tolerate oral medication.
- Oxycodone 5–10 mg PO available as needed.

Surgical Technique and Coordination in the Operating Room

The most consistent aspect of the same-day discharge program is the surgeon's technique. A surgeon's experience and comfort level performing the procedure definitely plays a role in operative time, soft tissue manipulation and trauma, and the ability to send people home on the same day. The surgery itself need not be rushed; even more critical is the communication and efficiency of the operative team. Surgical team members including physician assistants, nurses, and scrub techs need to be well-versed and facile in assisting the surgeon with the procedure, knowing the steps of the procedure, and how to facilitate efficient operating room turnover and set-up. The time between closure and incision of the subsequent case is where much of the time saving can be appreciated. The coordination of patient transfer, room turnover, and subsequent case set-up should run like a well-coordinated pit stop, where every member of the operating room team has a specific and consistent set of tasks. Tasks should be completed in parallel rather than in series: time should not be wasted waiting for one step to be completed before starting the next. As soon as the patient exits the operating room, the prior case instruments should already be removed from the room and the room cleaning and turnover started. As soon as instruments are verified as being available and in the room, the next patient should be entering the room to begin positioning and draping while the instruments are organized. The back table and mayo stands should be set up the same way each time so instruments are not missed and are easily located during the case. A sufficient number of instrument sets should be available to avoid sterile processing delays between cases. If feasible, a separate cart with all instruments individually peel-packed can be maintained as a backup to mitigate the inevitable processing issues or accidentally dropped instruments [13]. If the surgeon is using two operating rooms, each one should be an exact replica of the other to minimize delays or miscommunication and facilitate standardization. Timesaving on the order of minutes should be valued, where changes that create as little as a 5–10 min savings between each case can facilitate performing an additional case without added time to the day. Excellent surgical technique should not be compromised for the sake of time, and surgical time should not be the metric of operative time, but rather the time between drapes down to drapes up.

Postoperative Care and Physical Therapy

Preoperative counseling about the expectations for pain, as well as the intended use for each treatment, can empower patients to take control of their pain management after surgery, which will be required immediately as part of a same-day discharge. Explaining that pain and soreness during the first few days after surgery will be at their peak can normalize the experience and avoid psychologically induced escalation in pain leading to pain crisis and potential readmission or emergency room visits. Identifying, involving, and educating family and caregivers before surgery is important, as they become the primary nursing care for patients once they return home.

Once the patient arrives in the recovery area, acclimation after surgery should be seamless and quick. Perioperative nurses should be well-trained in specifically caring for same-day surgery patients and rapid recovery protocols including fluid hydration, pain control, and monitoring. The head of the bed should be raised to >50° immediately upon arrival. This helps reorient patients to their surroundings. Oxygen should be discontinued when saturation levels are above 92% on room air. Liquids should be started immediately to facilitate hydration and the diet should be advanced as tolerated. In the same way, oral pain medications should be started as soon as the patient is able to tolerate them. All of these measures attempt to encourage the patient that he or she is back to normalcy and not confined to the hospital bed with tubes and intravenous lines. Further, prolonged convalescence in bed should be avoided and the patient should be dressed in their clothing as soon as possible and transferred to a chair.

Physical therapy should be made aware of same-day surgery patients prior to the day of surgery so they can prioritize seeing them as soon as medically able. Patients who enter the operating room before noon may be more likely to go home on the same day compared with patients who have surgery after noon due to delay in mobilization and availability of time for therapy. Physical therapy should consult with the patient within 1–2 h after surgery if the anesthesia team uses an appropriately timed spinal. Timing of the spinal administration with the surgery is critical in making sure patients have return of motor function shortly after surgery and can participate in therapy without delay.

Physical therapy should focus on getting the patient to ambulate shortly after surgery. Again, this will simulate the home environment and encourage the patient that this is the normal postoperative protocol, rather than staying in bed. The goals for home discharge are below:

1. Walk 50–80 feet on level ground with minimal assistance.
2. Walk up and down stairs.
3. Perform bathroom transfers independently.
4. Go from a supine position in bed to standing.
5. Perform activities of daily living such as dressing oneself.
6. Understand how to perform exercises at home with and without assistance.

Medical Discharge Criteria

In addition to meeting the physical therapy goals noted above, the patient must meet the below medical criteria in order to be safely discharged home on the same day and avoid readmission:

1. Tolerate an oral diet.
2. No significant nausea or vomiting.
3. Void after surgery.
4. Pain well-controlled.
5. Vital signs stable.
6. Patient is seen and cleared by the operating surgeon.

Post-Discharge Follow-Up

Patients want to feel a constant connection with their surgeon and care team, especially if they are discharged home on the same day [14]. Patients often need to feel reassured that their pain level and swelling are within normal limits and their symptoms are all to be expected after surgery. Therefore, it is imperative to follow-up with the patient by phone within a week after surgery but preferably on postoperative day 1 to see how they are feeling. By reaching out early and establishing that the surgical team is available for the patient and able to normalize their experience, patients are more likely to feel at ease and report greater satisfaction with their recovery and care. As a result, patients may be less likely to go to the emergency room for issues that can be resolved over the phone with their surgeon or team [15].

Conclusion

As surgical technique and efficiency continue to improve and an emphasis shifts toward value-based healthcare, more and more arthroplasty surgeons will look to perform outpatient surgery. The ability to set up a comprehensive same-day surgery program involves the contributions and motivation of multiple parties, including the surgeon, anesthesia, surgical facility, and most importantly the patient. Surgeon leadership is paramount to success in aligning the goals of the hospital or surgery center with the surgeon. With clear leadership, standardized anesthesia, physical therapy, and recovery protocols can be put in place. Most importantly, recruiting appropriately screened and optimized patients for same-day surgery will result in the greatest chance of success. Consistent and deliberate counseling and care coordination prior to and throughout the surgical episode empower patients to take control of their recovery and ensures no detail is unclear or miscommunicated. Following these patients closely after surgery improves patient care, communication, and likely contributes to lower readmissions and greater satisfaction with the surgical process.

References

1. Fleischman AN, Austin MS, Purtill JJ, Parvizi J, Hozack WJ. Patients living alone can be safely discharged directly home after total joint arthroplasty: a prospective cohort study. J Bone Joint Surg Am. 2018;100(2):99–106.
2. Goyal N, Chen AF, Padgett SE, Tan TL, Kheir MM, Hopper RH, Hamilton WG, Hozack WJ. Otto Aufranc award: a multicenter, randomized study of outpatient versus inpatient total hip arthroplasty. Clin Orthop Relat Res. 2017;475(2):364–72.
3. Yoon RS, Nellans KW, Geller JA, Kim AD, Jacobs MR, Macaulay W. Patient education before hip or knee arthroplasty lowers length of stay. J Arthroplast. 2010;25(4):547–51.
4. Giraudet-Le Quintrec JS, Coste J, Vastel L, Pacault V, Jeanne L, Lamas JP, Kerboull L, Fougeray M, Conseiller C, Kahan A, Courpied JP. Positive effect of patient education for hip surgery: a randomized trial. Clin Orthop Relat Res. 2003;414:112–20.
5. Meneghini RM, Ziemba-Davis M, Ishmael MK, Kuzma AL, Caccavallo P. Safe selection of outpatient joint arthroplasty patients with medical risk stratification: the "outpatient arthroplasty risk assessment score". J Arthroplast. 2017;32(8):2325–31.
6. Ziemba-Davis M, Caccavallo P, Meneghini RM. Outpatient joint arthroplasty-patient selection: update on the outpatient arthroplasty risk assessment score. J Arthroplast. 2019;34(7S):S40–3.
7. Gogineni HC, Gray CF, Prieto HA, Deen JT, Boezaart AP, Parvataneni HK. Transition to outpatient total hip and knee arthroplasty: experience at an academic tertiary care center. Arthroplasty Today. 2019;5(1):100–5.
8. Turnbull ZA, Sastow D, Giambrone GP, Tedore T. Anesthesia for the patient undergoing total knee replacement: current status and future prospects. Local Reg Anesth. 2017;10:1–7.
9. Grosso MJ, Murtaugh T, Lakra A, Brown AR, Maniker RB, Cooper HJ, Macaulay W, Shah RP, Geller JA. Adductor canal block compared with periarticular bupivacaine injection for total knee arthroplasty: a prospective randomized trial. J Bone Joint Surg Am. 2018;100(13):1141–6.
10. Sardana V, Burzynski JM, Scuderi GR. Adductor canal block or local infiltrate analgesia for pain control after total knee arthroplasty? A systematic review and meta-analysis of randomized controlled trials. J Arthroplast. 2019;34(1):183–9.
11. Kulkarni MM, Dadheech AN, Wakankar HM, Ganjewar NV, Hedgire SS, Pandit HG. Randomized prospective comparative study of adductor canal block vs periarticular infiltration on early functional outcome after unilateral total knee arthroplasty. J Arthroplast. 2019;34(10):2360–4.
12. Eccles CJ, Swiergosz AM, Smith AF, Bhimani SJ, Smith LS, Malkani AL. Decreased opioid consumption and length of stay using an ipack and adductor canal nerve block following total knee arthroplasty. J Knee Surg. 2019;34:705.
13. Goldberg TD, Maltry JA, Ahuja M, Inzana JA. Logistical and economic advantages of sterile-packed, single-use instruments for total knee arthroplasty. J Arthroplast. 2019;34(9):1876–83.
14. Shah RP, Karas V, Berger RA. Rapid discharge and outpatient total joint arthroplasty introduce a burden of care to the surgeon. J Arthroplast. 2019;34(7):1307–11.
15. Sharareh B, Schwarzkopf R. Effectiveness of telemedical applications in postoperative follow-up after total joint arthroplasty. J Arthroplast. 2014;29(5):918–22.

Chapter 13
Staying Connected with the Patient after Discharge: Strategies and Resources

Tony S. Shen, Patawut Bovonratwet, and Michael P. Ast

Introduction

The demand for total joint arthroplasty (TJA) is projected to increase significantly in the coming decades [1]. As a result, the development of new strategies to maximize cost-effectiveness and to streamline the delivery of care is being increasingly explored. Outpatient arthroplasty has been shown to reduce the overall cost of surgery, largely by avoiding hospital admission [2]. A number of investigations into the safety of outpatient arthroplasty have been performed to date [3–7]. While comorbidities such as age greater than 80, smoking, bleeding disorders, and high ASA class were associated with an increased risk of complications, most studies conclude that outpatient arthroplasty is safe and cost-effective in carefully selected patients without clear risk factors for complication or readmission [8, 9].

In the outpatient setting, without the typical resources of the hospital in place, many elements of postoperative care rely on communication between the patient and the care team. A robust system of communication postoperatively plays a crucial role in minimizing unnecessary anxiety, reducing emergency room visits and readmissions, increasing patient satisfaction, and ultimately ensuring patient safety. A traditional hospital stay of several days allowed for several opportunities for patients to ask questions, have their anxiety alleviated, and have expectations set regarding normal occurrences after joint replacement surgery. The transition to outpatient surgery represents an important challenge and a potential opportunity for innovation. This chapter discusses strategies and resources for staying connected with outpatient TJA patients postoperatively.

T. S. Shen · P. Bovonratwet · M. P. Ast (✉)
Adult Reconstruction and Joint Replacement Service, Hospital for Special Surgery, New York, NY, USA
e-mail: shent@hss.edu; bovonratwetp@hss.edu; astm@hss.edu

R. M. Meneghini, L. T. Buller (eds.), *Outpatient Hip and Knee Replacement*,
https://doi.org/10.1007/978-3-031-27037-6_13

Options for Staying Connected

A traditional in-person follow-up visit is expensive and time-intensive for both the patient and surgeon and may not be the most cost-effective manner of communication postoperatively [10]. Marsh et al. showed that for the patient's first TJA follow-up visit in a traditional clinic setting, the cost to the healthcare payer perspective was approximately $71 while the cost to the societal perspective was $162 [11]. Due to advances in communications technology, other avenues of cost-effective patient follow-up are now being developed, including web-based assessments and HIPAA-compliant text messaging platforms. In the same study, Marsh et al. showed that for the patient's first TJA follow-up visit via a web-based assessment, the cost to the healthcare payer perspective was only $45 while the cost to the societal perspective was only $98 [11]. This difference in cost is an important consideration when designing an outpatient arthroplasty pathway with potentially more frequent postoperative communication.

Role of Telemedicine and Electronic-Based Follow-Up

Telemedicine originally referred to the use of information and communications technology to provide health services to people who are at a distance from their healthcare provider. However, due to the potential for substantial cost savings to the healthcare system, these methods have also been adapted to substitute for traditional in-person clinic follow-up visits [11]. Recent investigations of these technologically based follow-up strategies have demonstrated usefulness in monitoring recovery, reducing unplanned follow-up visits, and reducing costs.

Several types of nonconventional follow-up strategies utilizing communications technology have been reported in the literature. Hällfors et al. implemented a consultation telephone service for patients who underwent TJA and found that 87% of all issues were able to be resolved with a telephone conversation alone; the remaining 13% required further care in the emergency department [12]. In the context of outpatient arthroplasty, their results display an opportunity to optimize the strategy to safely address postoperative issues that may arise. While this area of study is relatively novel, there is an increasing body of literature reporting on the use of telemedicine and technologically based follow-up strategies.

Wood et al. described an electronic web-based assessment, where each patient was given a website address and a unique username/password to gain access to the web page and enter their data [13]. The web page could be accessed from any computer with an Internet connection. The web page contained the same questionnaires used in their outpatient clinic, with the exception of outcome scores that require physician input. Patient feedback at the conclusion of their study revealed that 95% of patients found the web assessment more convenient than a traditional clinic visit [13].

In another study by Sharareh et al., the authors utilized computer-based video conferencing software as their mode of follow-up with patients after TJA [14]. The live video sessions in their study were scheduled for 1 week, 3 weeks, 4 weeks, 6 weeks, and 9 weeks following surgery. All sessions consisted of a 30-min window. Outcome scores such as postoperative Hip Disability and Osteoarthritis Outcome Score (HOOS) and Knee Injury and Osteoarthritis Outcome Score (KOOS) were recorded for all patients undergoing total hip arthroplasty and total knee arthroplasty, respectively during these sessions [14]. After implementation of the live video program, the authors demonstrated a statistically significant reduction in unplanned clinic visits and calls. Additionally, the authors noted higher postoperative satisfaction in patients who underwent telemedicine follow-up compared to those who received traditional follow-up [14]. Similarly, positive results using video conferencing programs have also been reported in other non-arthroplasty settings [15, 16].

In addition to telephone or electronic communication, mobile-based patient engagement through smartphone applications (apps) has been explored with promising preliminary results [17]. Several of these exist in the orthopedic space, some of which were designed by their users and others that are commercially available through third-party vendors. Studies have been published with both of these types of mobile patient engagement platforms. Bitsaki et al. developed a mobile application that patients who underwent TJA can download on their smartphones. The mobile application in their study allows patients to fill in information about symptoms in the replaced joint and complete certain questionnaires (such as The Western Ontario and McMaster Universities Osteoarthritis Index). A cost analysis of their mobile-based system was notable for a total cost reduction of 13,578€ per patient [17].

Mobile-based patient engagement platforms not only facilitate patient communication and reduce costs but also have been shown to reduce unplanned hospital readmissions and postoperative complications. Rosner et al. demonstrated a reduction in potentially avoidable 90-day costs, 90-day hospital admissions, and complications after implementing a new class of automated digital patient engagement platforms, where patients received guidance and remote monitoring perioperatively. The investigators reviewed claims data for 186 patients enrolled in a digitally based follow-up program that was available online as well as on mobile devices. This group was compared to 372 patients who had traditional follow-up. They noted a mean savings of $656 per patient as well as a 54.4% relative reduction in postoperative complications [18]. Zhang et al. reviewed 1434 patients who were registered in an online follow-up platform. These patients were able to send images of their surgical wound for evaluation remotely. The investigators found that of the 430 patients who sent an image, 423 patients had normal-appearing wounds. The remaining patients were seen at a scheduled follow-up appointment [19].

In addition to patient monitoring, telemedicine and technologically based strategies may be used to augment postoperative rehabilitation. As a proof of concept, Russell et al. randomized patients who underwent primary total knee arthroplasty to 6 weeks of either conventional physical therapy or a simulated telerehabilitation program. The telerehabilitation group underwent their physical therapy session under the real-time guidance of a physical therapist through an Internet connection using only household equipment. These patients still traveled to the rehabilitation center and underwent their session in a standardized simulated living room with the physical therapist in another room. The investigators showed that outcomes achieved using telerehabilitation at 6 weeks following total knee arthroplasty were comparable with those after conventional rehabilitation. Patients in the telerehabilitation group also reported a high level of satisfaction [20]. Based on these results, Moffet et al. designed a trial in which total knee arthroplasty patients were randomized to true in-home telerehabilitation or traditional rehabilitation. They demonstrated that patient-reported outcomes (Western Ontario and McMaster Universities Osteoarthritis Index and Knee Injury and Osteoarthritis Outcome Score) in the in-home telerehabilitation group were non-inferior to those who underwent traditional rehabilitation [21].

Numerous additional studies have examined the utility of telerehabilitation in terms of clinical and economic effectiveness [22–24]. Other studies have investigated the validity of measurements made remotely in a telerehabilitation setting and found that the range of motion was highly reliable [25, 26]. In general, telerehabilitation has been shown to be noninferior to traditional in-person physical therapy for postoperative rehabilitation after TJA.

It is important to note however that just as the patient selection is critical for the safety of outpatient arthroplasty, not all patients are appropriate candidates for telerehabilitation. Klements et al. noted that approximately one-third of patients in their population benefited from traditional in-person therapy in addition to telerehabilitation [27, 28]. Further, Plate et al. reviewed the utilization pattern of their institutional electronic patient portal after TJA and found that patients who had risk factors for readmission such as discharge to an assisted living facility, Medicare/Medicaid insurance, and increased comorbidities were also less likely to use their electronic patient portal. Further, patients who did use the portal were found to have an increased readmission rate if the response rate to their messages was less than 75% [29].

Conclusion

As the landscape of TJA shifts towards the outpatient model, innovation in post-discharge patient communication may lead to improved patient satisfaction and cost-effectiveness. Technology-based patient communication platforms provide an opportunity to enhance postoperative care, as an increasing proportion of patients are likely to communicate using an online platform [30]. Already, orthopedic centers from around the world have reported promising results with remote patient monitoring and patient engagement platforms. When designing an outpatient arthroplasty pathway, the utilization of a technology-based patient engagement platform should be strongly considered to potentially decrease complications and readmissions and improve patient outcomes. Surgeons and team members can also choose to use these platforms to supplement postoperative physical therapy when appropriate.

References

1. Kurtz S, Ong K, Lau E, Mowat F, Halpern M. Projections of primary and revision hip and knee arthroplasty in the United States from 2005 to 2030. J Bone Joint Surg Ser A. 2007;89:780–5. https://doi.org/10.2106/JBJS.F.00222.
2. Huang A, Ryu JJ, Dervin G. Cost savings of outpatient versus standard inpatient total knee arthroplasty. Can J Surg. 2017;60:57–62. https://doi.org/10.1503/cjs.002516.
3. Bovonratwet P, Webb ML, Ondeck NT, Lukasiewicz AM, Cui JJ, McLynn RP, et al. Definitional differences of 'outpatient' versus 'inpatient' THA and TKA can affect study outcomes. Clin Orthop Relat Res. 2017;475:2917–25. https://doi.org/10.1007/s11999-017-5236-6.
4. Bovonratwet P, Ondeck NT, Tyagi V, Nelson SJ, Rubin LE, Grauer JN. Outpatient and Inpatient Unicompartmental Knee Arthroplasty Procedures Have Similar Short-Term Complication Profiles. J Arthroplast. 2017;32(10):2935–40. https://doi.org/10.1016/j.arth.2017.05.018.
5. Bovonratwet P, Ondeck NT, Nelson SJ, Cui JJ, Webb ML, Grauer JN. Comparison of outpatient vs inpatient total knee arthroplasty: an ACS-NSQIP. Analysis. 2017;32:1773. https://doi.org/10.1016/j.arth.2017.01.043.
6. Berger RA, Kusuma SK, Sanders SA, Thill ES, Sporer SM. The feasibility and perioperative complications of outpatient knee arthroplasty. Clin Orthop Relat Res. 2009;467:1443–9. https://doi.org/10.1007/s11999-009-0736-7.
7. Cross MB, Berger R. Feasibility and safety of performing outpatient unicompartmental knee arthroplasty. Int Orthop. 2014;38(2):443–7. https://doi.org/10.1007/s00264-013-2214-9.
8. Sher A, Keswani A, Yao DH, Anderson M, Koenig K, Moucha CS. Predictors of same-day discharge in primary total joint arthroplasty patients and risk factors for post-discharge complications. J Arthroplast. 2017;32:S150–S156.e1. https://doi.org/10.1016/j.arth.2016.12.017.
9. Courtney PM, Rozell JC, Melnic CM, Lee GC. Who should not undergo short stay hip and knee arthroplasty? Risk factors associated with major medical complications following primary total joint arthroplasty. J Arthroplast. 2015;30:1–4. https://doi.org/10.1016/j.arth.2015.01.056.
10. Koutras C, Bitsaki M, Koutras G, Nikolaou C, Heep H. Socioeconomic impact of e-health services in major joint replacement: a scoping review. Technol Health Care. 2015;23:809–17. https://doi.org/10.3233/THC-151036.
11. Marsh J, Hoch JS, Bryant D, MacDonald SJ, Naudie D, McCalden R, et al. Economic evaluation of web-based compared with in-person follow-up after total joint arthroplasty. J Bone Joint Surg Am. 2014;96:1910–6. https://doi.org/10.2106/JBJS.M.01558.
12. Hällfors E, Saku SA, Mäkinen TJ, Madanat R. A consultation phone service for patients with total joint arthroplasty may reduce unnecessary emergency department visits. J Arthroplast. 2018;33:650–4. https://doi.org/10.1016/j.arth.2017.10.040.
13. Wood G, Naudie D, MacDonald S, McCalden R, Bourne R. An electronic clinic for arthroplasty follow-up: a pilot study. Can J Surg. 2011;54:381–6. https://doi.org/10.1503/cjs.028510.
14. Sharareh B, Schwarzkopf R. Effectiveness of telemedical applications in postoperative follow-up after total joint arthroplasty. J Arthroplast. 2014;29:918–922.e1. https://doi.org/10.1016/j.arth.2013.09.019.
15. Good DW, Lui DF, Leonard M, Morris S, Mcelwain JP. Skype: a tool for functional assessment in orthopaedic research. J Telemed Telecare. 2012;18:94–8. https://doi.org/10.1258/jtt.2011.110814.

16. Armfield NR, Bradford M, Bradford NK. The clinical use of skype-for which patients, with which problems and in which settings? A snapshot review of the literature. Int J Med Inform. 2015;84:737–42. https://doi.org/10.1016/j.ijmedinf.2015.06.006.
17. Bitsaki M, Koutras G, Heep H, Koutras C. Cost-effective mobile-based healthcare system for managing total joint arthroplasty follow-up. Healthc Inform Res. 2017;23:67. https://doi.org/10.4258/hir.2017.23.1.67.
18. Rosner BI, Gottlieb M, Anderson WN. Effectiveness of an automated digital remote guidance and telemonitoring platform on costs, readmissions, and complications after hip and knee arthroplasties. J Arthroplast. 2017;33(4):988–996.e4. https://doi.org/10.1016/j.arth.2017.11.036.
19. Zhang J, Dushaj K, Rasquinha VJ, Scuderi GR, Hepinstall MS. Monitoring surgical incision sites in orthopedic patients using an online physician-patient messaging platform. J Arthroplast. 2019;34:1897–900. https://doi.org/10.1016/j.arth.2019.05.003.
20. Russell TG, Buttrum P, Wootton R, Jull GA. Internet-based outpatient telerehabilitation for patients following total knee arthroplasty: a randomized controlled trial. J Bone Joint Surg A. 2011;93:113–20. https://doi.org/10.2106/JBJS.I.01375.
21. Moffet H, Tousignant M, Nadeau S, Mérette C, Boissy P, Corriveau H, et al. In-home telerehabilitation compared with faceto-face rehabilitation after total knee arthroplasty: a noninferiority randomized controlled trial. J Bone Joint Surg Am. 2015;97:1129–41. https://doi.org/10.2106/JBJS.N.01066.
22. Jiang S, Xiang J, Gao X, Guo K, Liu B. The comparison of telerehabilitation and face-to-face rehabilitation after total knee arthroplasty: a systematic review and meta-analysis. J Telemed Telecare. 2018;24:257–62. https://doi.org/10.1177/1357633X16686748.
23. Fisher C, Biehl E, Titmuss MP, Schwartz R, Gantha CS. HSS@home, physical therapist-led telehealth care navigation for arthroplasty patients: a retrospective case series. HSS J. 2019;15:226–33. https://doi.org/10.1007/s11420-019-09714-x.
24. Chughtai M, Kelly J, Newman J, Sultan A, Khlopas A, Sodhi N, et al. The role of virtual rehabilitation in total and unicompartmental knee arthroplasty. J Knee Surg. 2019;32:105–10. https://doi.org/10.1055/s-0038-1637018.
25. Cabana F, Boissy P, Tousignant M, Moffet H, Corriveau H, Dumais R. Interrater agreement between telerehabilitation and face-to-face clinical outcome measurements for total knee arthroplasty. Telemed J E Health. 2010;16:293–8. https://doi.org/10.1089/tmj.2009.0106.
26. Shukla H, Nair S, Thakker D. Role of telerehabilitation in patients following total knee arthroplasty: evidence from a systematic literature review and meta-analysis. J Telemed Telecare. 2017;23:339–46. https://doi.org/10.1177/1357633X16628996.
27. Klement MR, Rondon AJ, McEntee RM, Kheir M, Austin MS. Web-based, self-directed physical therapy after total hip arthroplasty is safe and effective for most, but not all patients. J Arthroplast. 2019;34:513–6. https://doi.org/10.1016/j.arth.2018.10.032.
28. Klement MR, Rondon AJ, McEntee RM, Greenky MR, Austin MS. Web-based, self-directed physical therapy after Total knee arthroplasty is safe and effective for most, but not all, patients. J Arthroplast. 2019;34:S178–82. https://doi.org/10.1016/j.arth.2018.11.040.
29. Plate JF, Ryan SP, Bergen MA, Hong CS, Attarian DE, Seyler TM. Utilization of an electronic patient portal following total joint arthroplasty does not decrease readmissions. J Arthroplast. 2019;34:211–4. https://doi.org/10.1016/j.arth.2018.11.002.
30. Papas PV, Kim SJ, Ulcoq S, Cushner FD, Scuderi GR. The utilization of an internet-based patient portal and its impact on surgical outcomes in the TOTAL joint arthroplasty patient population. Orthop Proc. 2018;100-B:62. https://doi.org/10.1302/1358-992X.2018.12.062.

Chapter 14
Physical Therapy Following Same-Day Discharge Total Joint Arthroplasty

Matthew J. Grosso and William Hozack

Introduction

Along with other fields within total joint arthroplasty (TJA), physical therapy (PT) utilization has evolved significantly over the last decade. The tradition with regard to postoperative rehabilitation has been to administer formal guided PT to all patients undergoing TJA [1]. While the goals of therapy—to optimize return of function and allow for safe return to activities—have not changed over time, these goals were achieved primarily with inpatient PT, using strict discharge requirements, and often requiring a multiple-day hospital stay. In addition, a post-inpatient rehabilitation facility was promoted as an essential aspect of recovery following TJA [1].

With the advent of rapid recovery protocols, these paradigms have changed significantly, ultimately facilitating same-day discharge [2, 3]. Evidence-based medicine combined with an understanding of responsible resource management have greatly redefined the role of PT. For the modern same-day discharge TJA patient, a unique set of protocols are now in place that allow for safe and effective home discharge. Although the goals of safe and effective return to function are still similar, the timeline has shifted significantly, along with the methods to achieve these goals in same-day arthroplasty.

M. J. Grosso (✉) · W. Hozack
The Rothman Orthopaedic Institute & Thomas Jefferson University Hospital, Philadelphia, PA, USA
e-mail: william.hozack@rothmanortho.com

R. M. Meneghini, L. T. Buller (eds.), *Outpatient Hip and Knee Replacement*,
https://doi.org/10.1007/978-3-031-27037-6_14

Critical Factors for Successful Same-Day PT and Discharge

Same-day discharge is reliant on three critical factors that allow for postoperative mobilization with physical therapy: multimodal pain management, elimination of postoperative activity precautions, and reduced reliance on formal PT programs.

Same-day PT is critically dependent on an appropriate multimodal pain management protocol. At our institution, we follow a set protocol involving preoperative pain medications, minimization of opioid medications, peri-incisional injections, and regional nerve blocks. Preoperatively, patients receive oral acetaminophen (975 mg), pregabalin (75 mg), and celecoxib (400 mg) within 2 h of the surgical procedure. More recently, celecoxib is increasingly replaced with intravenous ketorolac (15 mg) given prior to incision. Postoperatively, standing doses of oral acetaminophen (650 mg) every 6 h, pregabalin (75 mg) every 12 h, and ketorolac (30 mg) every 6 h are administered to reduce reliance on breakthrough opioid medications [4]. Intraoperatively, peri-articular injections can be utilized in hip patients, but are more important for knee patients. A number of cocktails have been described, although ~60 mL of 0.5% bupivacaine has had success equivalent to more expensive cocktails, and currently is our standard of care [5]. In total knee arthroplasty patients, adductor canal blocks have demonstrated effectiveness in reducing pain and postoperative opioid consumption [6].

Elimination of postoperative precautions, particularly for total hip arthroplasty (THA), facilitates same-day PT and discharge. In a randomized controlled trial, Peak et al. demonstrated that utilization of functional restrictions following total hip arthroplasty does not reduce the prevalence of early postoperative dislocations [7]. This study examined dislocation rates utilizing an anterolateral approach, but similar reports have supported eliminating precautions for both the anterior and posterior approach as well [8, 9]. We believe that patients without precautions are less hesitant and more likely to mobilize both postoperatively, and post-discharge, allowing for more rapid recovery.

Finally, a critical factor necessary for successful same-day discharge is a reduced reliance on formal PT programs. The improved pain management regimens and reduced concerns about instability have created a situation in which outpatient TJA is a safe reality. In a prospective randomized trial, Goyal et al. randomized total hip arthroplasty (THA) patients to an outpatient (<12 h) versus inpatient (overnight, >12 h) stay. They demonstrated that outpatient care, including outpatient PT, led to similar outcomes, with no increase in complication rate [10]. In addition to same-day discharge, we discourage the utilization of inpatient rehabilitation. A number of studies have demonstrated no benefit, or even worse outcomes, with the utilization of post-discharge rehabilitation facilities [2, 11, 12]. We also emphasize outpatient PT over home PT. Outpatient PT requires mobilization out of the house, which has inherent value. A number of studies have demonstrated more rapid gains for patients who underwent outpatient PT compared to home PT following TKA [13, 14].

Role of Prehabilitation

Preoperative physical therapy sessions in preparation for surgery, or prehabilitation, have been considered for TJA patients. Evidence suggests that better preoperative health status (e.g., greater physical function and strength) is a predictor of good postoperative outcomes following TJA [15, 16]. Therefore, prehabilitation was introduced in an attempt to improve preoperative functional status, with the goal of improved postoperative outcomes. However, the current evidence is conflicting regarding the benefit of prehabilitation prior to TJA [17–20]. In a meta-analysis of 35 studies and 2956 patients, Moyer et al. reported that prehabilitation may result in small to moderate improvements in function and length of stay for both total hip and total knee patients, although the significant variety in preoperative exercises across studies made comparisons difficult [20]. At our institution, prehabilitation is not the standard of care and is reserved for a very small percentage of patients on a surgeon discretion basis. Patients receiving this prehabilitation program are rarely, if ever, being considered for same-day discharge. Further studies may be warranted to investigate the role of prehabilitation in improving rates of same-day discharge.

Day of Surgery Physical Therapy Protocols

Our institution follows a specific protocol for safe same-day discharge, for which physical therapy plays a critical role. Following surgery, PT is initiated within 1–6 h, with mean times closer to 1.5–3 h [10]. Since our patients have spinal anesthesia, initiation of PT can be delayed pending restoration of motor and sensory function. Modifications of the dosage and type of spinal anesthetic have facilitated this early mobilization. An appropriate multimodal pain management protocol, as discussed above, and close coordination with the anesthesia team are critical for early mobilization. Mobilization is achieved with the help of an assistive device, which can be crutches, walker, or a cane, depending on the patient, and physical therapist assessment. This device is usually the same device that the patient takes home. Once mobilized, there are a specific set of PT goals. In addition to medical and psychological factors, there are specific PT criteria that must be met prior to discharge, which include the ability to stand from a supine position in the bed, walk 80 feet, and go up and down stairs (Table 14.1). We find that these goals are

Table 14.1 Physical therapy discharge criteria for total joint arthroplasty

	Criteria
1.	Walk 80 feet on level ground
2.	Walk up and down stairs (if stairs at home)
3.	Demonstrate understanding of home exercises
4.	Perform bathroom transfers
5.	Stand from supine position in bed
6.	Be able to dress self and perform basic activities of daily living

achievable for the majority of patients. In a prospective cohort study from our institution, 26% of patients failed to achieve same-day discharge, but only a small portion of these patients (18% of failed-discharge patients, 5% of total cohort) failed because of inability to clear PT. [21]

These protocols are identical for total hip, total knee, and unicondylar knee replacement. For the total knee and unicondylar protocols, we also ensure patients understand the appropriate range-of-motion exercises, and inappropriate resting positions (such as a pillow under the leg).

Post-Discharge Physical Therapy Protocols

Traditionally, strict postoperative outpatient therapy has been administered to patients undergoing TJA. However, these paradigms have shifted, and there are several studies supporting no formal therapy for total hip arthroplasty, unicondylar knee arthroplasty, and select patients in total knee arthroplasty (TKA).

There is now strong evidence that suggests that formal PT is not required for the majority of patients who undergo THA. Austin et al. in a randomized controlled clinical trial, demonstrated that formal outpatient PT is not required following THA [22]. They report unsupervised home exercise is both safe and efficacious for a majority of patients. There are several alternatives to formal outpatient PT. Web-based, self-directed programs are gaining popularity and have shown efficacy in this population [23]. Group physiotherapy sessions are another alternative, which demonstrate efficiency and cost-effectiveness [24]. However, it is the authors' preference to avoid any formalized protocol, and, instead, to emphasize to the patient to perform their normal daily activities, and that each of those activities requires movement of the hip. This is discussed with the patients as a customized PT program based on activities of daily living.

The issue of formal PT is more complex following TKA, because of a greater concern for early range of motion postoperatively. Failure to achieve degrees of flexion and extension can lead to limitations in daily activities and poor outcomes [25, 26]. Laubenthal et al. demonstrated that 67° of flexion is needed for the swing phase of gait, 83° for climbing stairs, 90° for descending stairs, and 93° for standing up from a chair [25]. Therefore, we have been more hesitant in eliminating formal PT in our total knee arthroplasty patients. However, Fleischman et al. demonstrated that unsupervised home exercise is not inferior to outpatient PT after TKA [27]. They demonstrated a similar range of motion and patient-reported outcomes through 6 months postoperatively. To ensure success, patient selection can be critical. Wang and colleagues showed that an early postoperative visit (approximately 2 weeks) may be helpful to identify patients who are not progressing appropriately and can benefit from formal PT. [28] Web-based protocols may also help decrease the number of patients who require formal therapy sessions [29].

While range of motion is still a concern following unicondylar knee arthroplasty (UKA), it is less of an issue compared to TKA [30]. Similar to THA, evidence suggests that the majority of UKA patients do well with self-directed exercises following UKA. In a randomized clinical trial comparing formal outpatient PT to unsupervised home exercises, Fillingham et al. demonstrated no differences in ROM or patient reported outcomes at 6 weeks from surgery [31]. However, of the 25 patients randomized to the unsupervised therapy, three (12%), crossed over to the formal outpatient PT group due to limited progress. This suggests that a subset of UKA patients may not be suitable for unsupervised therapy, and further work is needed to identify the at-risk cohort.

For those patients requiring post-discharge PT, as stated in the critical factors section, our preference is for post-discharge outpatient PT over home PT. We see significant value in the act of mobilizing to the outpatient PT center, which requires mobility, transfers, and knee ROM at multiple time points (in and out of car, staircases, walking across the street, etc.). Indeed, a number of studies have demonstrated more rapid gains for patients who underwent outpatient PT compared to home PT following TKA [13, 14].

Conclusions

Postoperative physical therapy has evolved with rapid recovery protocols to allow safe and effective same-day discharge following primary TJA. Immediate postoperative therapy (POD0) should focus on early mobilization and meeting discharge goals in a safe and effective manner. Post-discharge formal physical therapy is not required for most patients who undergo outpatient joint replacement surgery. Defining the appropriate patients suitable for unsupervised home exercise programs is critical, particularly for total knee arthroplasty patients.

References

1. Naylor JM, Hart A, Mittal R, Harris IA, Xuan W. The effectiveness of inpatient rehabilitation after uncomplicated total hip arthroplasty: a propensity score matched cohort. BMC Musculoskelet Disord. 2018;19:236. https://doi.org/10.1186/s12891-018-2134-3.
2. Buhagiar MA, Naylor JM, Harris IA, Xuan W, Kohler F, Wright R, et al. Effect of inpatient rehabilitation vs a monitored home-based program on mobility in patients with total knee arthroplasty: the HIHO randomized clinical trial. JAMA. 2017;317:1037–46. https://doi.org/10.1001/jama.2017.1224.
3. Abdul-Hadi O, Hozack WJ. The rapid recovery program for total hip arthroplasty. In: Surgical treatment of hip arthritis: reconstruction, replacement & revision. Philadelphia, PA: Saunders Elsevier; 2009, p. 225–231.

4. Fleischman AN, Tarabichi M, Foltz C, Makar G, Hozack WJ, Austin MS, et al. Cluster-randomized trial of opiate-sparing analgesia after discharge from elective hip surgery. J Am Coll Surg. 2019;229:335–345.e5. https://doi.org/10.1016/j.jamcollsurg.2019.05.026.
5. Grosso MJ, Murtaugh T, Lakra A, Brown AR, Maniker RB, Cooper HJ, et al. Adductor canal block compared with periarticular bupivacaine injection for total knee arthroplasty: a prospective randomized trial. J Bone Joint Surg Am. 2018;100:1141–6. https://doi.org/10.2106/JBJS.17.01177.
6. Beausang DH, Pozek J-PJ, Chen AF, Hozack WJ, Kaufmann MW, Torjman MC, et al. A randomized controlled trial comparing adductor canal catheter and intraarticular catheter after primary total knee arthroplasty. J Arthroplast. 2016;31:298–301. https://doi.org/10.1016/j.arth.2016.01.064.
7. Peak EL, Parvizi J, Ciminiello M, Purtill JJ, Sharkey PF, Hozack WJ, et al. The role of patient restrictions in reducing the prevalence of early dislocation following total hip arthroplasty. A randomized, prospective study. J Bone Joint Surg Am. 2005;87:247–53. https://doi.org/10.2106/JBJS.C.01513.
8. Restrepo C, Mortazavi SMJ, Brothers J, Parvizi J, Rothman RH. Hip dislocation: are hip precautions necessary in anterior approaches? Clin Orthop Relat Res. 2011;469:417–22. https://doi.org/10.1007/s11999-010-1668-y.
9. Kornuijt A, Das D, Sijbesma T, van der Weegen W. The rate of dislocation is not increased when minimal precautions are used after total hip arthroplasty using the posterolateral approach: a prospective, comparative safety study. Bone Joint J. 2016;98-B:589–94. https://doi.org/10.1302/0301-620X.98B5.36701.
10. Goyal N, Chen AF, Padgett SE, Tan TL, Kheir MM, Hopper RH, et al. Otto Aufranc award: a multicenter, randomized study of outpatient versus inpatient total hip arthroplasty. Clin Orthop Relat Res. 2017;475:364–72. https://doi.org/10.1007/s11999-016-4915-z.
11. Mahomed NN, Davis AM, Hawker G, Badley E, Davey JR, Syed KA, et al. Inpatient compared with home-based rehabilitation following primary unilateral total hip or knee replacement: a randomized controlled trial. J Bone Joint Surg Am. 2008;90:1673–80. https://doi.org/10.2106/JBJS.G.01108.
12. Chimenti CE, Ingersoll G. Comparison of home health care physical therapy outcomes following total knee replacement with and without subacute rehabilitation. J Geriatr Phys Ther. 2007;30:102–8. https://doi.org/10.1519/00139143-200712000-00004.
13. Warren M, Kozik J, Cook J, Prefontaine P, Ganley K. A comparative study to determine functional and clinical outcome differences between patients receiving outpatient direct physical therapy versus home physical therapy followed by outpatient physical therapy after total knee arthroplasty. Orthop Nurs. 2016;35:382–90. https://doi.org/10.1097/NOR.0000000000000295.
14. Christensen JC, Paxton RJ, Baym C, Forster JE, Dayton MR, Hogan CA, et al. Benefits of direct patient discharge to outpatient physical therapy after total knee arthroplasty. Disabil Rehabil. 2019;42:1–7. https://doi.org/10.1080/09638288.2018.1505968.
15. Fortin PR, Clarke AE, Joseph L, Liang MH, Tanzer M, Ferland D, et al. Outcomes of total hip and knee replacement: preoperative functional status predicts outcomes at six months after surgery. Arthritis Rheum. 1999;42:1722–8. https://doi.org/10.1002/1529-0131(199908)42:8<1722::AID-ANR22>3.0.CO;2-R.
16. Ethgen O, Bruyère O, Richy F, Dardennes C, Reginster JY. Health-related quality of life in total hip and total knee arthroplasty. A qualitative and systematic review of the literature. J Bone Joint Surg Am. 2004;86:963–74. https://doi.org/10.2106/00004623-200405000-00012.
17. Gill SD, McBurney H. Does exercise reduce pain and improve physical function before hip or knee replacement surgery? A systematic review and meta-analysis of randomized controlled trials. Arch Phys Med Rehabil. 2013;94:164–76. https://doi.org/10.1016/j.apmr.2012.08.211.
18. Ackerman IN, Bennell KL. Does pre-operative physiotherapy improve outcomes from lower limb joint replacement surgery? A systematic review. Aust J Physiother. 2004;50:25–30. https://doi.org/10.1016/s0004-9514(14)60245-2.

19. Wallis JA, Taylor NF. Pre-operative interventions (non-surgical and non-pharmacological) for patients with hip or knee osteoarthritis awaiting joint replacement surgery–a systematic review and meta-analysis. Osteoarthr Cartil. 2011;19:1381–95. https://doi.org/10.1016/j.joca.2011.09.001.
20. Moyer R, Ikert K, Long K, Marsh J. The value of preoperative exercise and education for patients undergoing total hip and knee arthroplasty: a systematic review and meta-analysis. JBJS Rev. 2017;5:e2. https://doi.org/10.2106/JBJS.RVW.17.00015.
21. Fraser JF, Danoff JR, Manrique J, Reynolds MJ, Hozack WJ. Identifying reasons for failed same-day discharge following primary total hip arthroplasty. J Arthroplast. 2018;33:3624–8. https://doi.org/10.1016/j.arth.2018.08.003.
22. Austin MS, Urbani BT, Fleischman AN, Fernando ND, Purtill JJ, Hozack WJ, et al. Formal physical therapy after total hip arthroplasty is not required: a randomized controlled trial. J Bone Joint Surg Am. 2017;99:648–55. https://doi.org/10.2106/JBJS.16.00674.
23. Klement MR, Rondon AJ, McEntee RM, Kheir M, Austin MS. Web-based, self-directed physical therapy after total hip arthroplasty is safe and effective for most, but not all, patients. J Arthroplast. 2019;34:513–6. https://doi.org/10.1016/j.arth.2018.10.032.
24. Coulter CL, Weber JM, Scarvell JM. Group physiotherapy provides similar outcomes for participants after joint replacement surgery as 1-to-1 physiotherapy: a sequential cohort study. Arch Phys Med Rehabil. 2009;90:1727–33. https://doi.org/10.1016/j.apmr.2009.04.019.
25. Laubenthal KN, Smidt GL, Kettelkamp DB. A quantitative analysis of knee motion during activities of daily living. Phys Ther. 1972;52:34–43. https://doi.org/10.1093/ptj/52.1.34.
26. Huddleston J, Alaiti A, Goldvasser D, Scarborough D, Freiberg A, Rubash H, et al. Ambulatory measurement of knee motion and physical activity: preliminary evaluation of a smart activity monitor. J Neuroeng Rehabil. 2006;3:21. https://doi.org/10.1186/1743-0003-3-21.
27. Fleischman AN, Crizer MP, Tarabichi M, Smith S, Rothman RH, Lonner JH, et al. 2018 John N. Insall award: recovery of knee flexion with unsupervised home exercise is not inferior to outpatient physical therapy after TKA: a randomized trial. Clin Orthop Relat Res. 2019;477:60–9. https://doi.org/10.1097/CORR.0000000000000561.
28. Wang WL, Rondon AJ, Tan TL, Wilsman J, Purtill JJ. Self-directed home exercises vs outpatient physical therapy after total knee arthroplasty: value and outcomes following a protocol change. J Arthroplast. 2019;34:2388–91. https://doi.org/10.1016/j.arth.2019.05.020.
29. Russell TG, Buttrum P, Wootton R, Jull GA. Internet-based outpatient telerehabilitation for patients following total knee arthroplasty: a randomized controlled trial. J Bone Joint Surg Am. 2011;93:113–20. https://doi.org/10.2106/JBJS.I.01375.
30. Kleeblad LJ, van der List JP, Zuiderbaan HA, Pearle AD. Larger range of motion and increased return to activity, but higher revision rates following unicompartmental versus total knee arthroplasty in patients under 65: a systematic review. Knee Surg Sports Traumatol Arthrosc. 2018;26:1811–22. https://doi.org/10.1007/s00167-017-4817-y.
31. Fillingham YA, Darrith B, Lonner JH, Culvern C, Crizer M, Della Valle CJ. Formal physical therapy may not be necessary after unicompartmental knee arthroplasty: a randomized clinical trial. J Arthroplast. 2018;33:S93–S99.e3. https://doi.org/10.1016/j.arth.2018.02.049.

Chapter 15
Strategies to Minimize Patient Anxiety, Emergency Room Visits, and Readmissions Following Outpatient Total Joint Arthroplasty

Charles De Cook

Introduction

Already the highest expenditure in the CMS budget, total joint arthroplasty (TJA) utilization is projected to rise exponentially over the coming decades, especially across younger patient demographics [1]. At the same time, the rise in value-based payment models has brought tremendous emphasis on healthcare cost containment. The convergence of these trends makes the successful reduction in the length of hospital (LOS) stay after TJA both crucial and feasible. Indeed, over the last 30 years, the average LOS after TJA, particularly after total knee arthroplasty (TKA) and total hip arthroplasty (THA), has gone from a few weeks to a few days, and now to a same-day procedure in the ambulatory surgery setting. But 30/90-day readmissions of Medicare beneficiaries after TJA surgery have been reported to be as high as 15% [2, 3]. Reducing LOS is only meaningful when we concurrently reduce (or eliminate) avoidable emergency room (ER) visits and hospital readmissions postsurgery.

The patient's state of mind going into surgery is an often under-appreciated factor in postsurgical outcomes [4]. Minimizing patient anxiety prior to surgery leads to better outcomes, including a reduction in avoidable ER visits and readmissions (Fig. 15.1). Thus, anxiety reduction methods through effective patient engagement and education are key component of a successful preoperative patient preparation strategy.

C. De Cook (✉)
Total Joint Specialists, Atlanta, GA, USA

R. M. Meneghini, L. T. Buller (eds.), *Outpatient Hip and Knee Replacement*,
https://doi.org/10.1007/978-3-031-27037-6_15

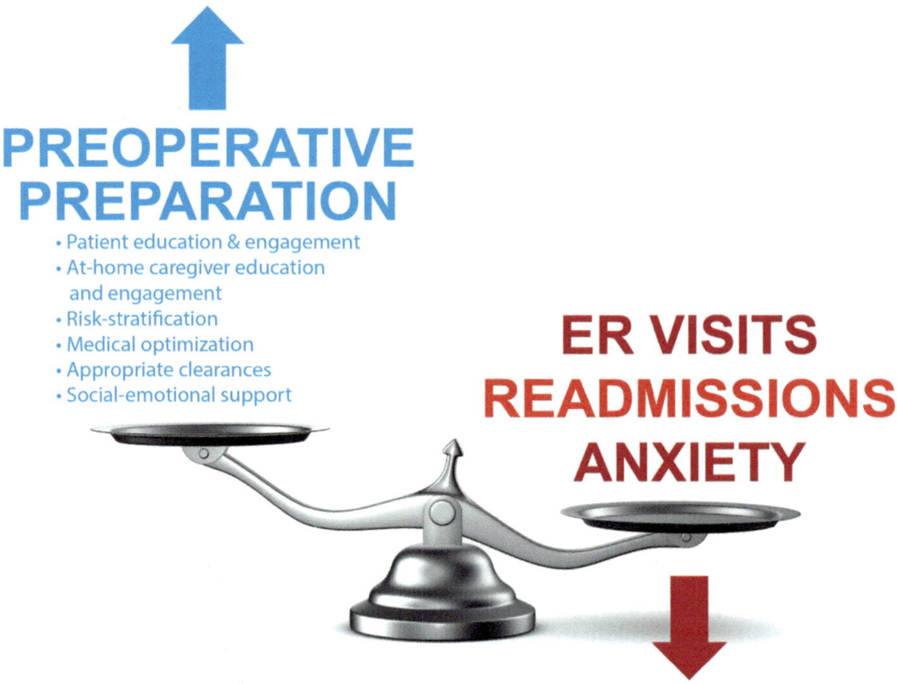
PREOPERATIVE
PREPARATION
• Patient education & engagement
• At-home caregiver education and engagement
• Risk-stratification
• Medical optimization
• Appropriate clearances
• Social-emotional support
ER VISITS
READMISSIONS
ANXIETY

Fig. 15.1 When preoperative preparation goes up, anxiety, ER visits, and hospital readmissions during recovery go down

Anxiety and Patient Outcomes

It is common for people to experience anxiety when anticipating surgery. A significant part of patient anxiety comes from not knowing what to expect during or after the operation. Patients typically harbor unknowns about anesthesia, separation from family, postoperative pain, loss of independence, and changes in body image [5]. When will they be able to walk again? When will they be able to drive? Will they be able to go to the washroom by themselves? When can they resume normal activities? When will they return to work?

Placebo-controlled studies have taught us how strong the placebo effect can be, especially for a surgical procedure, [6] demonstrating that what patients believe preoperatively about their surgery directly impacts what they believe postoperatively about their outcome. Unfortunately, minimizing patient anxiety is not a common priority of current preoperative preparation. Patients are frequently left in the dark and can feel abandoned, particularly when it comes to the day of surgery [7]. Add to that the long wait times usually associated with TJA surgery, and patients may spend weeks or months trapped in a negative anxiety loop, predisposing them to poor outcomes before their surgery even begins.

Reducing Patient Anxiety

Alleviating preoperative anxiety is, of course, a mental game. Patient anxiety is best addressed prospectively, with formal protocols for the entire care team around active listening and dispelling patient "unknowns" through effective engagement and education (Fig. 15.2). Patients do better when they are encouraged from the beginning to play an active role in their own preoperative preparation and feel less anxious when they have a sense of when they will be able to get back to their normal activities after surgery.

One strategy that has been shown to be successful toward reducing patient anxiety is to demonstrate empathy [8]. When patients feel that they have been listened to, they feel understood and validated. This means that we must not only provide patients with educational content but should encourage patients to express their emotions and share any questions they have, preferably in person. Done properly, this approach can transform the typically stressful process of obtaining appropriate

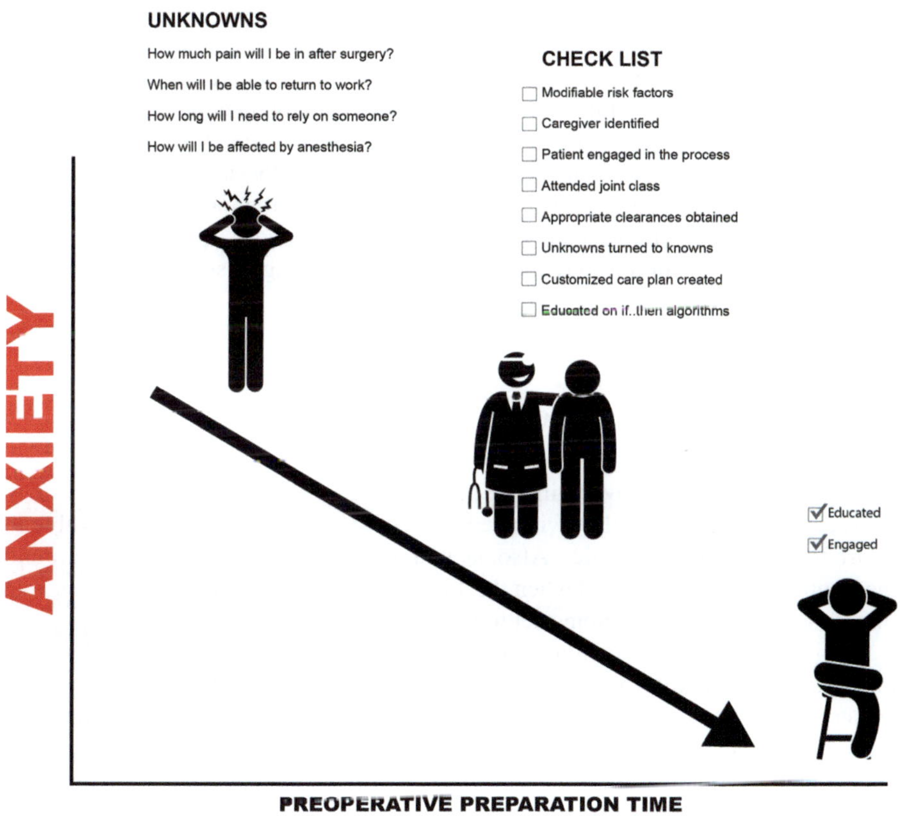

Fig. 15.2 Systematically engaging and educating patients as part of preoperative preparation changes their "unknowns" to "knowns" and minimizes anxiety

clearances into a more copacetic experience. Multiple experiments [9] have shown that a deliberately supportive patient-practitioner relationship is key to creating belief in a successful outcome.

The first office visit is the best time to understand each patient's goals for their TJA surgery and to set their expectations on positive outcomes. This can help the patient maintain the perspective that it is their choice to have this surgery and ensure that the whole care team understands what the patient is aiming to achieve. Ask enabling questions during this visit, such as "Who is going to take care of you after surgery?" This serves not only the practical purpose of ensuring there is an adequate postsurgery plan in place but also engages the patient early on in visualizing a successful postoperative arrangement in which their needs are being met. Another way of doing this is to introduce patients before surgery to some of the physical therapy exercises they will be given during their postoperative recovery, so they gain a sense of what these motions look and feel like before surgical pain and dysfunction set in. When a patient's needs, goals, and modifiable risk factors are identified up front, the whole care team can work together to ensure that the patient's preoperative preparation is aligned accordingly.

The fear of being unconscious has been shown to be a significant cause of anxiety for patients on the day of surgery [10]. It is common for patients to experience "anesthetic catastrophizing," which is the fear of being rendered unconscious and not waking up, of dying while under the anesthetic, of having a mask put over their face, and of having to put their trust in strangers. A recent survey showed that 20% of patients were worried about brain damage from anesthesia, waking up during surgery, and having memory loss, while roughly half that amount (9%) were concerned about postoperative pain [11]. With concerns about anesthesia being so widespread, it is important to reduce anxiety by dispelling misconceptions associated with regional or general anesthesia.

Reducing Caregiver Anxiety

Like the patient, the caregiver will also be faced with unknowns regarding what they will need to do, how long they will need to do it, and when they, too, will be able to return to their normal activities. Also, as with the patient, caregiver anxiety around these unknowns is heightened when the TJA is performed at an ASC, with their role of caring for the patient at home set to begin the same day as the surgery.

Similar to reducing patient anxiety, caregiver anxiety is best addressed by turning unknowns into knowns at the outset through effective presurgery education and engagement. The sooner the caregiver understands their role, the better. The caregiver, who is generally a family member, friend, neighbor, or coworker, should be encouraged to attend all meetings and classes with the patient, as well as attending a class designed especially for caregivers of patients after TJA surgery [12]. Caregivers should be made to feel like the critical stakeholder they are throughout all relevant aspects of preoperative risk assessment and preparation. They should also be encouraged to embrace the social-emotional aspect of their role such as partnering with the patient to set expectations before surgery around positive post-surgery outcomes.

Reducing Surgeon Anxiety

ASCs are safe economical settings for TJA surgeries [13]. However, performing TJAs at ASCs is more logistically complex relative to performing TJAs in the hospital setting. Traditional hospital settings offer a wealth of space, equipment, and support staff, backed by a long history of established procedures for addressing any complication that may arise during or after surgery. In contrast, ASCs are designed for efficiency, such that surgeons who come sufficiently prepared in advance have everything they need, and nothing extra [14]. This makes meticulous preoperative patient selection and preparation more than "nice-to-have"; it is essential. Postoperative adverse events such as heart attacks, sleep apnea, anemia, or respiratory arrest are less of a concern when the patient is staying the night in the hospital and can be managed and monitored by healthcare professionals. Hence, surgeons who are relatively new to performing TJAs at ASCs may experience some heightened preoperative anxiety of their own.

Surgeons can minimize their own anxiety by making sure to have rigorous patient selection and medical optimization processes in place and by creating the right team culture. When implementing complex and life-dependent yet mundane processes, Atul Gawande advocates using a checklist [15]. One critical component of a successful presurgery preparation process is making sure everyone knows who is in charge of patient optimization. Further, surgeon anxiety will be minimized when it is allowed to be normalized within a deliberate care team culture. Surgeons should be expected to bring their "A" game every day, but at the same time feel comfortable letting their team know when a particular patient or procedure may be cause for extra concern, paving the way for their team to then give that particular patient or procedure the extra attention that is needed.

ER Visits and Hospital Readmissions

People spend more time in the hospital today than at any other time in history [16]. And, the number of patients who bounce back to the hospital shortly after being discharged can be significant. Combined 30-day readmission rates for THA and TKA procedures are around 4.4% [17]. A meta-analysis of readmission rates published between 1982 and 2013 found that for THA, rates are 5.6% at 30 days and 7.7% at 90 days, while for TKA, rates are 3.3% at 30 days and 9.7% at 90 days [18].

It might be expected that performing TJAs in the ASC setting carries an inherently higher risk of ER visits and readmissions during recovery. This is a misconception. Between 2004 and 2008, when joint replacements happened exclusively in the hospital setting with a typical LOS of 3–5 days [19], there was actually a dramatic increase in readmission rates of Medicare patients within 90 days of THA (primary or revision), from 7.4% to 11.9% [20]. Ninety day readmission rates following TKA over the same time period were even higher, at 15.6% [2]. This puts a strain on the healthcare system, making the elimination of preventable ER visits and hospital readmissions a priority for policymakers. In addition to the financial burden, avoidable hospital visits expose patients to undue risks of nosocomial and iatrogenic infections. Perhaps most importantly, ER visits and hospital readmissions carry an incalculable emotional toll on patients and their loved ones.

Reducing ER Visits

The reality is that patients who undergo TJA surgery at an ASC are less likely to experience catastrophic complications, including a cardiac event and pulmonary embolism (PE), than those who have the procedure performed in a traditional hospital setting [21]. This is a testament to the power of proper preoperative preparation and patient selection, whereby we select low-risk patients and engage in effective patient education and medical optimization prior to surgery. Minimization of unnecessary ER visits during recovery is a hallmark of success in the outpatient arena. The more prepared patients and caregivers are before surgery, the easier it is for patients to gain solid footing on the road to a smooth recovery after surgery because they understand what to expect.

The most common reasons for postoperative ER visits are pain, swelling, and/or medication side effects [22, 23]. Common causes of ER visits among older patients are fluid and electrolyte disorders. Evidence is mounting that teaching patients how to detect early signs of these issues and proactively address them before they escalate results in less futile use of the ER. Arming patients and caregivers in advance with appropriate "if … then" statements prior to surgery will minimize the likelihood of these things leading to ER visits. "If you experience swelling, then you should …," or "If your wound becomes red, then you should … ".

Reducing Readmissions

Another assumption that might seem reasonable is the notion that the more time TJA patients get to spend recovering in the hospital after surgery, the better their outcomes. In fact, longer lengths of postsurgery hospital stays for TJA patients, particularly stays over 3 days, have been shown to correlate with a higher likelihood of postoperative complications and readmissions [24].

When it comes to readmission following TJA surgery, the rates are lower than that of the general Medicare population but still significant. The most common reason for postoperative TJA readmissions is surgical site infection. These readmissions can happen at unpredictable times [25] and they pose a financial burden to hospitals under the bundled healthcare payment model [26].

In a study of 5732 patients undergoing either THA or TKA between 2013 and 2018, it was revealed that the major risk factors associated with readmissions are age, body mass index (BMI), smoking, narcotic use, length of stay, discharge to skilled nursing facility and multiple comorbidities, such as psychiatric diagnoses and occurrence of cardiac dysrhythmias [27]. These risk factors were similar for both 30-day and 90-day readmissions. Clearly, the key to predicting, and potentially avoiding, readmission after surgery lies in performing comprehensive risk assessments prior to surgery. This enables us to preemptively identify risk factors that can be modified prior to surgery, such as working with patients to lower their BMI, stop smoking, stop using narcotics and get treatment for psychiatric disorders.

If a patient is shown to be at high risk of complications due to modifiable factors, it is important to delay TJA surgery long enough to optimize that patient. Improving one or more of these risk factors will directly impact the likelihood of hospital readmission after surgery. Multiple studies have shown that with appropriate patient selection, arthroplasty patients can be discharged safely on the same day as surgery [21]. One way to take advantage of modifiable risk factors and extended preoperative patient care is to make use of preoperative optimization programs. Such programs have been shown to reduce complications, such as readmission, after TJA [28].

Another common misconception is the perceived benefit of sending patients to skilled nursing facilities, rather than sending them home. In fact, it has been shown that complications and readmission rates are higher if you send patients to a skilled nursing facility versus sending them home [29]. As long as your care team works closely with the patient and their at-home caregiver, providing adequate education and decreasing modifiable risk factors ahead of surgery, sending TJA patients home the same day is the best option.

Patients who are candidates for TJA in the ASC setting must be assessed upfront for the level of social support from family and friends that will be available to them after surgery. One patient will have a spouse and older children at home to help with postoperative care, while another patient might live alone. One patient will have good mental health, while another might struggle with addiction and depression. Studies of TJAs performed in the hospital setting have shown that the greater the social support that patients receive from family and friends postsurgery, the lower the patient's length of stay. Conversely, the higher a patient's psychological distress and the less social support they have, the longer their length of stay is likely to be. However, even with higher psychological distress, higher social support will still result in a shorter length of stay [30].

Useful Tools for Reducing Anxiety, ER Visits, and Readmissions

Apps for Patients and Caregivers

Traditionally, patients and caregivers have been instructed to page the provider on-call should urgent concerns arise. These traditional interactions between patients and healthcare providers tend to be information-heavy, but short in terms of time [31]. They can also produce varied success. Fortunately, today there are medical apps that are designed with patient-centered care in mind. This technology helps a healthcare team connect with and monitor patients who are comfortable communicating via apps on their smartphones or mobile technologies [32].

With the right assistive apps, patients can, in theory, engage in an integrated care pathway that follows them through all stages of their TJA experience, from the initial referral through surgery and recovery. These apps can provide patients with targeted educational materials and customized care plans, potentially saving patients from getting misinformed by following the wrong sources online. Ideally, these apps can also collect patient-reported outcomes on symptoms, medication side effects, and even levels of postsurgical anxiety or distress and link these patient inputs to provider alerts. This model offers an efficient way to preemptively address patient concerns and provide comprehensive care coordination, while the patient is still at home and *before* the issues escalate into avoidable ER visits.

Assessment Tools for Surgeons

Simply knowing the risk factors is not enough. Once the data is gathered, it must be iteratively modified and reassessed to achieve target patient optimization. This is a complex process. Fortunately, there are preoperative evidence-based assessment tools that can be used to help determine not only the risk factors involved with a patient's TJA surgery but how those risk factors might affect the outcome and post-operative recovery.

The first tool is the Readmission Risk Assessment Tool (RRAT) [33]. This is a tool that should be applied to all clinical, referral, preoperative, and surgical information regarding the patient. The RRAT allows a patient's healthcare team to analyze their data and develop a risk stratification that identifies the number and severity of modifiable risks the patient has. Once the RRAT score has been calculated, the patient can be identified as high-risk or low-risk for readmission.

Another assessment tool that is useful for a TJA patient's healthcare team is the Outpatient Arthroplasty Risk Assessment (OARA). This assessment tool is a validated multidisciplinary algorithm for risk stratification and patient assessment that was designed specifically for the identification of patients for both same-day and next-day discharge after TJA surgery [34]. The assessment is geared toward the safety of the patient, with scores between 0 and 79 identifying patients who are good candidates for day surgery. Patients are scored on the basis of nine health categories, which include general health, hematology, cardiology, endocrine, gastrointestinal, renal, pulmonary, psychiatric/neurological, and infectious disease [35].

Conclusion

By 2030, the overall number of total knee arthroplasties (TKA) and total hip arthroplasties (THA) are expected to reach 3.48 million and 572,000 respectively [36, 37]. When it comes to TJA in the outpatient setting, preparation is the key to success and for reducing postoperative ER visits and readmissions. Patients often experience heightened anxiety prior to surgery, and if a patient is at high risk for complications, this can increase the anxiety of everyone involved, including the patient, the caregiver, the surgeon, and the healthcare team. It is absolutely critical that, as surgeons, we understand a patient's individual risk factors, both modifiable and those that are not. Of particular importance are the modifiable risk factors, which include obesity, poor nutrition, poorly controlled diabetes, smoking, venous thromboembolic disease, cardiovascular disease, and psychological and neurocognitive problems, behavioral problems, *Staphylococcus aureus* colonization, physical deconditioning and the risk of falling. These risk factors have been proven to negatively affect postoperative outcomes and increase the risk of readmission [38].

It is critically important to consider comorbidities ***prior*** to surgical intervention, as this has been shown to reduce postsurgical complications and improve outcomes. When this is coupled with the medical optimization of high-risk TJA candidates, it also improves patient engagement, which, in turn, reduces anxiety. An example of this is Perioperative Orthopedic Surgical Home (POSH), which is an optimization pathway that targets eight modifiable comorbidities that were targeted by the RRAT and are identified by surgeon-led screening [39]. These include infection risks; smoking; obesity/malnutrition; cardiovascular disease; deep venous thrombosis; neurocognitive, psychological, or substance-related problems; physical deconditioning; diabetes.

As technology continues to improve and patient-centered care is fully embraced, patients will feel increasingly listened to, understood, and validated. This will result in a better understanding of the TJA surgical procedure and the postoperative outcome. The key is to initiate this patient education early in the preoperative stages of the care pathway, so the patient has time to learn and digest information, have their questions and concerns addressed, and form relationships with their healthcare team. When this happens consistently and thoroughly, patient preoperative anxiety will be significantly reduced, which will in turn reduce the likelihood of postoperative ER visits and readmissions (Fig. 15.3).

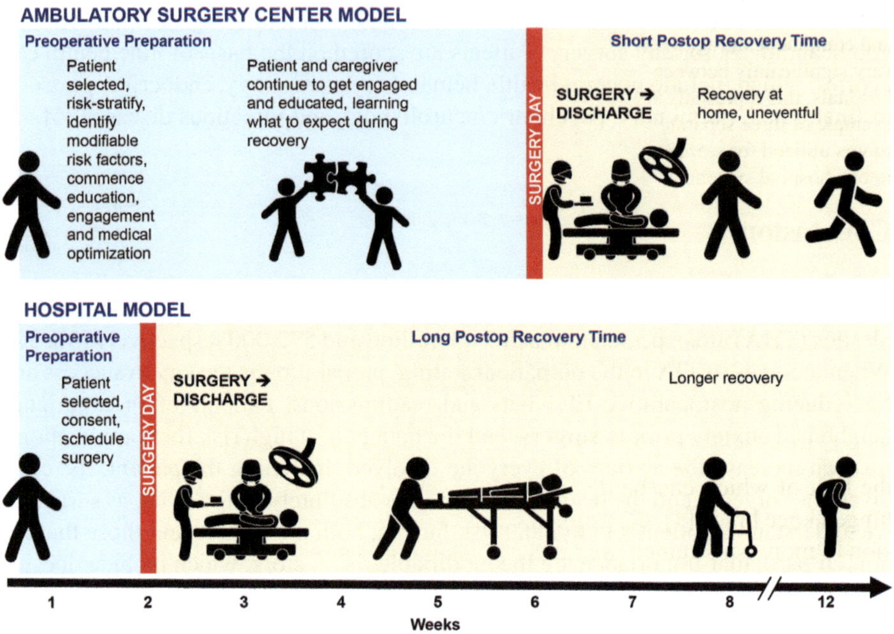

Fig. 15.3 Total joint arthroplasty patient experience at an ambulatory surgery center versus the hospital setting

References

1. Molloy IB, Martin BI, Moschetti WE, Jevsevar DS. Effects of the length of stay on the cost of total knee and total hip arthroplasty from 2002 to 2013. J Bone Joint Surg Am. 2017;99(5):402–7.
2. Husted H, Otte KS, Kristensen BB, Orsnes T, Kehlet H. Readmissions after fast-track hip and knee arthroplasty. Arch Orthop Trauma Surg. 2010;130(9):1185–91.
3. Hoffmann JD, Kusnezov NA, Dunn JC, Zarkadis NJ, Goodman GP, Berger RA. The shift to same-day outpatient joint arthroplasty: a systematic review. J Arthroplast. 2018;33(4):1265–74.
4. Alattas SA, Smith T, Bhatti M, Wilson-Nunn D, Donell S. Greater pre-operative anxiety, pain and poorer function predict a worse outcome of a total knee arthroplasty. Knee Surg Sports Traumatol Arthrosc. 2017;25(11):3403–10.
5. Bailey L. Strategies for decreasing patient anxiety in the perioperative setting. AORN J. 2010;92(4):445–57.
6. Carroll EE. The placebo effect doesn't apply just to pills. The New York Times; October 6, 2014. https://www.nytimes.com/2014/10/07/upshot/the-placebo-effect-doesnt-apply-just-to-pills.html.
7. Gilmartin J, Wright K. Day surgery: patients' felt abandoned during the preoperative wait. J Clin Nurs. 2008;17(18):2418–25.
8. Pereira L, Figueiredo-Braga M, Carvalho IP. Preoperative anxiety in ambulatory surgery: the impact of an empathic patient-centered approach on psychological and clinical outcomes. Patient Educ Couns. 2016;99(5):733–8.
9. Vance E. Unlocking the healing power of you. National Geographic; 2016. https://www.nationalgeographic.com/magazine/2016/12/healing-science-belief-placebo/.
10. Mitchell M. General anaesthesia and day-case patient anxiety. J Adv Nurs. 2010;66(5):1059–71.

11. Matthey P, Finucane BT, Finegan BA. The attitude of the general public towards preoperative assessment and risks associated with general anesthesia. Can J Anaesth. 2001;48(4):333–9.
12. Edwards PK, Mears SC, Lowry BC. Preoperative education for hip and knee replacement: never stop learning. Curr Rev Musculoskelet Med. 2017;10(3):356–64.
13. Shah RR, Cipparrone NE, Gordon AC, Raab DJ, Bresch JR, Shah NA. Is it safe? Outpatient total joint arthroplasty with discharge to home at a freestanding ambulatory surgical center. Arthroplast Today. 2018;4(4):484–7.
14. Davis KK, Mahishi V, Singal R, Urman RD, Miller MA, Cooke M, et al. Quality improvement in ambulatory surgery centers: a major national effort aimed at reducing infections and other surgical complications. J Clin Med Res. 2019;11(1):7–14.
15. Gawande A. The checklist manifesto: how to get things right. New York: Metropolitan Books; 2009.
16. Gwande A. Being mortal: medicine and what matters in the end: metropolitan books. New York: Henry Hold and Company; 2014.
17. Ramaswamy A, Marchese M, Cole AP, Harmouch S, Friedlander D, Weissman JS, et al. Comparison of hospital readmission after total hip and total knee arthroplasty vs spinal surgery after implementation of the hospital readmissions reduction program. JAMA Netw Open. 2019;2(5):e194634.
18. Ramkumar PN, Chu CT, Harris JD, Athiviraham A, Harrington MA, White DL, Berger DH, Naik AD, Li LT. Causes and rates of unplanned readmissions after elective primary total joint arthroplasty: a systematic review and meta-analysis. Am J Orthop (Belle Mead NJ). 2015;44(9):397–405.
19. Lam V, Teutsch S, Fielding J. Hip and knee replacements: a neglected potential savings opportunity. JAMA. 2018;319(10):977–8.
20. Cram P. Clinical characteristics and outcomes of medicare patients undergoing total hip arthroplasty, 1991-2008. JAMA. 2011;305(15):1560.
21. Johnson DJ, Hartwell MJ, Weiner JA, Hardt KD, Manning DW. Which postoperative day after total joint arthroplasty are catastrophic events most likely to occur? J Arthroplast. 2019;34(10):2466–72.
22. Sibia US, Mandelblatt AE, Callanan MA, MacDonald JH, King PJ. Incidence, risk factors, and costs for hospital returns after total joint arthroplasties. J Arthroplast. 2017;32(2):381–5.
23. Kelly MP, Prentice HA, Wang W, Fasig BH, Sheth DS, Paxton EW. Reasons for ninety-day emergency visits and readmissions after elective total joint arthroplasty: results from a US integrated healthcare system. J Arthroplast. 2018;33(7):2075–81.
24. Otero JE, Gholson JJ, Pugely AJ, Gao Y, Bedard NA, Callaghan JJ. Length of hospitalization after joint arthroplasty: does early discharge affect complications and readmission rates? J Arthroplast. 2016;31(12):2714–25.
25. Dailey EA, Cizik A, Kasten J, Chapman JR, Lee MJ. Risk factors for readmission of orthopaedic surgical patients. J Bone Joint Surg Am. 2013;95(11):1012–9.
26. Phillips JLH, Rondon AJ, Vannello C, Fillingham YA, Austin MS, Courtney PM. How much does a readmission cost the bundle following primary hip and knee arthroplasty? J Arthroplast. 2019;34(5):819–23.
27. Greiwe RM, Spanyer JM, Nolan JR, Rodgers RN, Hill MA, Harm RG. Improving orthopedic patient outcomes: a model to predict 30-day and 90-day readmission rates following total joint arthroplasty. J Arthroplast. 2019;34(11):2544–8.
28. Cyriac J, Garson L, Schwarzkopf R, Ahn K, Rinehart J, Vakharia S, et al. Total joint replacement perioperative surgical home program: 2-year follow-up. Anesth Analg. 2016;123(1):51–62.
29. Owens JM, Callaghan JJ, Duchman KR, Bedard NA, Otero JE. Short-term morbidity and readmissions increase with skilled nursing facility discharge after total joint arthroplasty in a medicare-eligible and skilled nursing facility-eligible patient cohort. J Arthroplast. 2018;33(5):1343–7.
30. Zeppieri KE, Butera KA, Iams D, Parvataneni HK, George SZ. The role of social support and psychological distress in predicting discharge: a pilot study for hip and knee arthroplasty patients. J Arthroplast. 2019;34(11):2555–60.

31. van Kasteren Y, Freyne J, Hussain MS. Total knee replacement and the effect of technology on cocreation for improved outcomes and delivery: qualitative multi-stakeholder study. J Med Internet Res. 2018;20(3):e95.
32. Semple JL, Armstrong KA. Mobile applications for postoperative monitoring after discharge. CMAJ. 2017;189(1):E22–4.
33. Boraiah S, Joo L, Inneh IA, Rathod P, Meftah M, Band P, et al. Management of modifiable risk factors prior to primary hip and knee arthroplasty: a readmission risk assessment tool. J Bone Joint Surg Am. 2015;97(23):1921–8.
34. Ziemba-Davis M, Caccavallo P, Meneghini RM. Outpatient joint arthroplasty-patient selection: update on the outpatient arthroplasty risk assessment score. J Arthroplast. 2019;34(7S):S40–3.
35. International Congress for Joint Reconstruction. Selecting patients for outpatient surgery: a novel scoring system. February 25, 2019. https://icjr.net/articles/selecting-patients-for-outpatient-surgery-a-novel-scoring-system.
36. Kurtz S, Ong K, Lau E, Mowat F, Halpern M. Projections of primary and revision hip and knee arthroplasty in the United States from 2005 to 2030. J Bone Joint Surg Am. 2007;89(4):780–5.
37. Sloan M, Premkumar A, Sheth NP. Projected volume of primary total joint arthroplasty in the U.S., 2014 to 2030. J Bone Joint Surg Am. 2018;100(17):1455–60.
38. Yu S, Garvin KL, Healy WL, Pellegrini VD Jr, Iorio R. Preventing hospital readmissions and limiting the complications associated with total joint arthroplasty. J Am Acad Orthop Surg. 2015;23(11):e60–71.
39. Kim KY, Anoushiravani AA, Chen KK, Li R, Bosco JA, Slover JD, et al. Perioperative orthopedic surgical home: optimizing total joint arthroplasty candidates and preventing readmission. J Arthroplast. 2019;34(7S):S91–6.

Chapter 16
Making the Transition to Outpatient: Resources and Pathway Changes

Paul K. Edwards, Jeffrey B. Stambough, Simon C. Mears, and C. Lowry Barnes

Introduction

Making the transition to outpatient (OP) total hip and knee replacement can have many challenges. Recently, surgeons have sought to identify the critical steps to accomplish this transition [1–7]. Our total joint arthroplasty (TJA) clinical pathway (CP) is a structured, multidisciplinary plan of care, with detailed steps that are standardized to elective total hip and knee replacement patients. This chapter identifies some of the key elements in a successful CP that we recommend initiating prior to an OP TJA program.

Patient Selection

Appropriate patient selection combined with proper preoperative optimization is vital to the success of an OP TJA program. Recent reports have shown that utilizing strict OP exclusion criteria results in similar risks of adverse events and readmissions between OP and inpatient (IP) TJA. Excluding patients with a history of diabetes mellitus, myocardial infarction, stroke, congestive heart failure, deep venous thromboembolism, pulmonary embolism, cardiac arrhythmia, respiratory failure, chronic pain requiring regular opioid medications, active cardiopulmonary disease, history of sleep apnea, active anticoagulation therapy, and morbid obesity from OP selection yields similar outcomes to inpatient TJA [8–10].

P. K. Edwards (✉) · J. B. Stambough · S. C. Mears · C. L. Barnes
Orthopaedic Surgery, University of Arkansas for Medical Sciences, Little Rock, AR, USA
e-mail: jstambough@uams.edu; scmears@uams.edu; clbarnes@uams.edu

R. M. Meneghini, L. T. Buller (eds.), *Outpatient Hip and Knee Replacement*,
https://doi.org/10.1007/978-3-031-27037-6_16

An increased risk in perioperative TJA complications has been reported in patients age >75 years, uncontrolled diabetes, chronic obstructive pulmonary disease, high BMI (>35 kg/m^2), chronic opioid use, functional neurological impairments, dependent functional status, low preoperative cognitive capacity, congestive heart failure, liver cirrhosis, and chronic kidney disease [11–13]. Other institutions have implemented thresholds for outpatient TJA for candid consideration including BMI < 35 kg/m^2, ASA classification <3, strong social support system with an available "coach" for the first 2 postoperative weeks, <75 years of age, and able to participate in an outpatient program [13, 14]. The partners in our total joint practice have agreed upon a few strict exclusion criteria for OP TJA (Table 16.1).

Table 16.1 Exclusion criteria for outpatient TJA

Medical Factors	Psychosocial Factors
CHF	Age > 70 years
CVA	Live alone
CKD	History of falls
ESRD	Excessive alcohol/drug abuse
COPD	Smoking history
Hepatitis	Chronic opioid use
HIV/AIDS	History of depression/anxiety
Sleep apnea	Assistance for ADLs
BMI >40 kg/m^2	Lack of transportation
Atrial fibrillation	Chronic pressure ulcers
Vascular disease	Hospitalization <6 months ago
Chornic steroid use	Admission to SNF <6 months ago
History of post-op ileus	Noncompliance with home meds
Solid organ transplant	No "coach" or caretaker
CAD with prior cardiac stents	
Chronic anemia (Hgb <10 g/dL)	
Thrombocytopenai (platelets <75 k)	
ASA = > 4 assessed by anesthesia	
History of malignant hyperthermia	
Malnutrition	
*Total lymphocytes <1500 cells/mm	
*Albumin <3.5 g/dL	
Transferrin level < 200 mg/dL	

Preoperative Optimization/Clearance Pathways

Utilization of two distinct medical clearance pathways are beneficial. One pathway is reserved for patients that are healthier and can be considered potentially appropriate for OP TJA, while the second pathway includes patients with more extensive medical issues (e.g., uncontrolled hypertension, pulmonary issues, congestive heart failure, prior cardiac stents, coagulopathies, prior DVT/PE, anticoagulation agents beyond ASA, chronic anemia, end-stage renal disease, etc.) [2]. Patients are initially screened by the surgeon or mid-level provider at the surgical office visit. Relatively healthy patients along with those meeting OP TJA criteria are referred to one of our three fellowship-trained Sports Medicine Primary Care Physician (PCP) partners to undergo a thorough medical evaluation. We have learned that a single location for medical optimization/clearance provides many benefits and minimizes preoperative clearance variability. While this streamlined process not only provides a single depot for history, physical exams, and consultant medical clearances (e.g., Cardiology, Hematology, etc.), it also affords consistent and judicious use of preoperative medical laboratory studies that aligns with our overarching goal of providing a safe, cost-conscious approach for joint replacement. The patients who do not meet OP criteria are referred to our Internal Medicine (IM) colleagues for further evaluation/optimization dependent on their comorbidities. Patients referred to the IM pathway are *not* candidates for OP TJA.

Education

Preoperative hip and knee replacement education classes are paramount to successful short stay joint replacement. These sessions have demonstrated utility in decreasing pre- and postoperative anxiety, postoperative pain, improving coping skills, leading to shorter length of stay (LOS), improving home discharge, lowering readmissions, and imparting cost savings to the episode of care [1, 6, 7, 15–28]. Specifically, implementation of a CP with a mandatory preoperative educational program has demonstrated shorter hospital LOS, decreased readmissions, and improved home discharge [1, 2, 5–7]. Recent data revealed preoperative education as the single intervention associated with decreasing LOS following total knee arthroplasty without increasing complications or readmissions within 90 days of discharge [28].

One key feature to improve learning and retention is the use of general information tailored to the specific procedure in an interactive format using the "*spaced retention method*" [29–31]. A previous review article outlines this method as effective in educating adult patients regarding their elective hip or knee replacement surgery. This technique has been shown to increase memory retention by up to 200% [32–34]. Our CP accomplishes this teaching by aligning the surgeon, surgeon's mid-level provider, surgeon's office RN, PCP Sports Medicine Clearance team, and the preoperative education instructors to teach consistent, correct detailed information in repetition at varying spaced intervals.

In addition to proper preoperative education, it is vital that the education material is written at a level the patient can comprehend. Since only 12% of US adults have proficient health literacy, patient education material should be written at a sixth grade or lower reading level and include pictures and illustrations [35, 36]. It is important to note the patient education material provided by the American Academy of Orthopaedic Surgeons (AAOS) has a readability score above the eighth grade level and therefore may need to be modified or tailored to some of your patient population [37–41]. Presenters should be the treating staff and classes should be taught on or near the joint replacement hospital floor [20]. Other guidelines for the preoperative education material suggest avoiding medical jargon, structuring the program to be chronological, and using visual images and models for demonstration [20].

Perhaps an even more critical element to successful OP TJA is the identification of a strong support system [42]. We require our OP TJA candidates to have a family member or close friend, designated as a "coach," commit to being available as a caretaker for at least 2 weeks after surgery and to assist the patient on the day of discharge. It is important to educate the patient and their "coach" to pay special attention to warning signs that could indicate a medical complication that can occur in the first 24 h after a procedure, such as oversedation, urinary retention, nausea, vomiting, dehydration, and hypotension. Therefore, we require *mandatory* patient attendance and highly encourage "coach" attendance for the educational joint academy class prior to elective hip or knee arthroplasty. Our patients also sign a "non-binding" contract in which they identify their "coach" as well as three individuals available to assist with personal needs and transportation after hospital discharge (Figs. 16.1 and 16.2). If a patient fails to attend class, we delay surgery until the class can be completed. For complete transparency and partner accountability, our practice emails a monthly report that details the percentage of each surgeon's patients and coaches who attend the education class prior to joint replacement.

UAMS
Department of Orthopaedic Surgery

UAMS HIPKNEE ACADEMY AGREEMENT

Welcome to the UAMS HipKnee Academy. Our goal is to give you the information you need to have the best experience you can with your replacement surgery. We aim to send you home with family or friends the day after surgery. We do not plan to send you to inpatient rehab, skilled nursing home, or home health unless medically needed.

What we do:

- Keep pain under control
- Use long acting numbing shots
- Help you to walk the day of surgery
- Help you to get home and to move around as quickly as possible
- Start physical therapy the day after knee patients leave the hospital
- Help patients stay out of rehabs where they could get infections

What is not usally needed:

- IV narcotic drugs
- Urinary catheters
- IV lines
- Long hospital stays
- Continuous passive motion machines (CPMs) because they have not been shown to help patients
- Physical therapy for hip patients

We need to make sure you understand our program and have the support of family and friends you need to recover. **Please bring this signed form with you to the HipKnee Academy class at UAMS.**

I agree to attend HipKnee Academy at UAMS. This class will help me to understand what to expect with my surgery, when I go home, and therapy. I do not have to attend if I have been to HipKnee Academy in the last year.

I agree to bring my coach with me to HipKnee Academy. This coach is someone who will be with me at home for the first five to seven days after surgery.

I agree to see a doctor at UAMS before my surgery.

I agree to use the phone numbers that will be given to me if I need medical help. I will be given a daytime phone number to call during clinic hours, and a separate phone number for nights or weekends to reach a doctor or physician assistant (PA). I will call these numbers instead of going to my primary care clinic or the emergency room first. I will call those numbers if I have trouble with pain, swelling, redness, or am worried about infection.

Figs. 16.1 and 16.2 Total joint arthroplasty patient contract

UAMS
Department of Orthopaedic Surgery

By signing this form, I agree to the above and understand that I must plan to follow all discharge instructions from my surgeon. If I do not do all that I have agreed to, my surgery may be rescheduled or cancelled.

______________________________ ______________

Patient Signature Date

My coach will be ______________________.

The following people will be able to help with my personal needs and driving after I leave the hospital:

____
____
____
____
____

Thank you for choosing UAMS for your joint replacement suregery. We look forward to giving you the best care before, during, and after your surgery. See you in HipKnee Academy!

Sincerely,
UAMS Hip and Knee Replacement team

Simon C. Mears, M.D., Ph.D.
Paul K. Edwards, M.D.
C. Lowry Barnes, M.D.
Jeffrey B. Stambough, M.D.

Figs. 16.1 and 16.2 (continued)

Anesthesia

Modern neuraxial spinal anesthesia (SA) has been the preferred anesthetic modality for rapid recovery in elective TJA. Several studies from high-volume joint replacement centers have reported SA is associated with less blood loss, lower transfusions rates, shorter LOS, lower rates of intensive care unit (ICU) utilization, lower rates of cardiopulmonary complications, lower deep vein thrombosis risks, and improved 30-day morbidity and mortality [43–47]. Although SA remains the accepted standard for OP TJA, recent reports show that excellent outcomes can be achieved when modern general anesthetic (GA) techniques are utilized. We recently reported equivocal complications and outcomes using contemporary GA techniques in a series of 1527 consecutive primary TJAs (644 total hip and 883 total knee arthroplasties) performed over a 3-year span at a single institution. In our cohort, 96.3% of patients were discharged in less than 24 h after elective TJA with a 2.4% 90-day readmission rate and a 1.3% reoperation rate [48]. Our contemporary GA techniques are detailed in this recent publication [48].

Same-Day Discharge Criteria

Once a patient has been determined as a potential candidate for OP TJA surgery, it is important to adequately inform the patient and family of the risks and potential benefits of same-day discharge. The patient, their "coach," and their support team should understand the same-day discharge criteria and agree to participate in this pathway. If surgery is performed in a free-standing Ambulatory Surgery Center, there needs to be previously established protocols with efficient pathways in place to allow for IP hospital admission in the circumstance when same-day discharge criteria are not met.

Recently, AAHKS proposed evidence-based guidelines be followed for safe same-day discharge to home after TJA (http://www.aahks.org/position-statements/outpatient-joint-replacement/). Prior to discharge, all patients should undergo a comprehensive physical therapy evaluation. Patients should be able to ambulate with assistance to and from the bathroom, ascend and descend at least two steps, and walk independently on ground level using an assistive device. Patients should demonstrate they can tolerate oral fluids, have pain controlled with oral medications, void without difficulty, and remain hemodynamically stable (Table 16.2). Systematic processes at all centers participating in OP TJA must be in place to allow for such changes in care plans if an IP admission is necessary. The conditions listed in Table 16.3 need to be assessed carefully and if they place the patient at increased risk for complications or adverse events, then IP admission should occur (Table 16.3).

Table 16.2 Same-day TJA discharge criteria

Social support network in place
Voids without difficulty
Tolerates oral fluids without difficulty
Adequate pain control with oral medications
Remains hemodynamically stable during mobilization
Physical therapy requirement
*Safely ambulate
*Independently transfer
*Ascend/descend steps

Table 16.3 Appropriate TJA inpatient admission criteria

Requires assistance of PT to safely ambulate
Home environment not conducive to safe recovery
Requires monitoring of electrolytes or hematologic parameters
Requires monitoring of medical condition (diabetes, hypertension, etc.)
Unable to understand postoperative instructions (precautions, medication adherence, or safety)
Any other condition or status that is likely to require a level of support, intervention, or monitoring not readily available outside of the hospital inpatient setting
Existence of any one of the following factors:
*Inadequate pain control on oral pain medication
*Unable to tolerate oral intake
*Unable to void freely
*Hemodynamically unstable

Staying Connected

Communication after home discharge is critical to safe and successful outcomes. In an effort to avoid unnecessary Emergency Department (ED) visits, office visits, and hospital readmissions all patients are instructed to call a "hotline" number for any questions or concerns. We also counsel all patients to call the "hotline" prior to making any unplanned visit to the ED. Patient calls during daytime hours are received by our office nursing staff and addressed with the respective team. After-hours and weekend questions are addressed via the "hotline" number that is answered by a rotating schedule of one of the surgeons or mid-level providers. A recent study has shown that managing an all access number is actually not as burdensome as one may imagine. Our data showed on average one phone call was received per day, with an average duration of 3.9 min per call [49].

In addition to the patient "hotline" number, we contract with a third-party group to assist in proactive patient phone calls at specific pre- and postoperative intervals. The purpose of these calls is to identify and solve any issues or patient concerns prior to an unnecessary ED visit, readmission, or office visit. These "touches" allow for real-time clinical decision-making and for an adjustment in the frequency of "touches" depending on the severity of the particular issues. In concert with our clinical pathway, we have previously demonstrated excellent outcomes with very low complication and readmission rates through the different phases of care.

References

1. Edwards PK, Levine M, Cullinan K, Newbern G, Barnes CL. Avoiding readmissions-support systems required after discharge to continue rapid recovery? J Arthroplast. 2015;30(4):527–30.
2. Edwards PK, Barnes CL. Dealing with the outliers—physicians, inpatient post-acute care providers, physical therapists, and visiting nursing facilities. Semin Arthroplast. 2016:27(3).
3. Althausen PL, Mead L. Bundled payments for care improvement: lessons learned in the first year. J Orthop Trauma. 2016;30(Suppl 5):S50–3.
4. Iorio R, Bosco J, Slover J, Sayeed Y, Zuckerman JD. Single institution early experience with the bundled payments for care improvement initiative. J Bone Joint Surg Am. 2017;99(1):e2.
5. Berend KR, Lombardi AV, Mallory TH. Rapid recovery protocol for peri-operative care of total hip and total knee arthroplasty patients. Surg Technol Int. 2004;13:239–47.
6. MacDonald V, Arthur B, Parent S. The Vancouver general hospital joint replacement rapid recovery program: optimizing outcomes through focused pathways. J Orthop Nurs. 2005;9:95–102.
7. Pennington JM, Jones DPG, McIntyre S. Clinical pathways in total knee arthroplasty. A New Zealand experience. J Orthop Surg. 2003;11:165–73.
8. Kolisek FR, McGrath MS, Jessup NM, Monesmith EA, Mont MA. Comparison of outpatient versus inpatient total knee arthroplasty. Clin Orthop Relat Res. 2009;467(06):1438–42.
9. Berger RA, Sanders S, Gerlinger T, Della Valle C, Jacobs JJ, Rosenberg AG. Outpatient total knee arthroplasty with a minimally invasive technique. J Arthroplast. 2005;20(07, Suppl 3):33–8.

10. Springer BD, Odum SM, Vegari DN, Mokris JG, Beaver WB Jr. Impact of inpatient versus outpatient total joint arthroplasty on 30-day hospital readmission rates and unplanned episodes of care. Orthop Clin North Am. 2017;48(01):15–23.
11. Rozell JC, Courtney PM, Dattilo JR, Wu CH, Lee GC. Late complications following elective primary total hip and knee arthroplasty: who, when, and how? J Arthroplast. 2017;32(03):719–23.
12. Courtney PM, Boniello AJ, Berger RA. Complications following outpatient total joint arthroplasty: an analysis of a national database. J Arthroplast. 2017;32(5):1426–30. https://doi.org/10.1016/j.arth.2016.11.055. Epub 2016 Dec 14.
13. Kort NP, Bemelmans YFL, van der Kuy PHM, Jansen J, Schotanus MGM. Patient selection criteria for outpatient joint arthroplasty. Knee Surg Sports Traumatol Arthrosc. 2017;25(09):2668–75.
14. Argenson JN, Husted H, Lombardi A Jr, Booth RE, Thienpont E. Global forum: an international perspective on outpatient surgical procedures for adult hip and knee reconstruction. J Bone Joint Surg Am. 2016;98(13):e55.
15. Edwards PK, Mears SC, Barnes CL. BPCI: everyone wins, including the patient. J Arthroplast. 2017;32(6):1728–31.
16. Crowe J, Henderson J. Pre-arthroplasty rehabilitation is effective in reducing hospital stay. Can J Occup Ther. 2003;70:88–96.
17. Kelly MH, Ackerman M. Total joint arthroplasty: a comparison of past acute settings on patient functional outcomes. Orthop Nurs. 1999;18:75–84.
18. Daltroy LH, Morlino CI, Eaton HM, Poss R, Liang MH. Preoperative education for total hip and knee replacement patients. Arthritis Care Res. 1998;11:469–78.
19. Sjoling M, Nordahl G, Olofsson N, Asplund K. The impact of preoperative information on state anxiety, postoperative pain and satisfaction with pain management. Patient Educ Couns. 2003;51:169–76.
20. Spalding NJ. Reducing anxiety by pre-operative education: make the future familiar. Occup Ther Int. 2003;10:278–93.
21. Lin PC, Lin LC, Lin JJ. Comparing the effectiveness of different educational programs for patients with total knee arthroplasty. Orthop Nurs. 1997;16:43–9.
22. Butler GS, Hurley CA, Buchanan KL, Smith-VanHorne J. Prehospital education: effectiveness with total hip replacement surgery patients. Patient Educ Couns. 1996;29:189–97.
23. Bondy LR, Sims N, Schroeder DR, Offord KP, Narr BJ. The effect of anesthetic patient education on preoperative patient anxiety. Reg Anesth Pain Med. 1999;24:158–64.
24. Giraudet-Le Quintrec JS, Coste J, Vastel L, Pacault V, Jeanne L, Lamas JP, et al. Positive effect of patient education for hip surgery: a randomized trial. Clin Orthop Relat Res. 2003;1:112–20.
25. Gammon J, Mulholland CW. Effect of preparatory information prior to elective total hip replacement on post-operative physical coping outcomes. Int J Nurs Stud. 1996;33:589–604.
26. Moulton LS, Evans PA, Starks I, Smith T. Pre-operative education prior to elective hip arthroplasty surgery improves postoperative outcome. Int Orthop. 2015;39(8):1483–6.
27. Tait MA, Dredge C, Barnes CL. Preoperative patient education for hip and knee arthroplasty: financial benefit? J Surg Orthop Adv. 2015;24(4):246–51.
28. Jones S, Alnaib M, Kokkinakis M, Wilkinson M, St Clair Gibson A, Kader D. Pre-operative patient education reduces length of stay after knee joint arthroplasty. Ann R Coll Surg Engl. 2011;93:71–5.
29. Luck A, Pearson S, Maddern G, Hewett P. Effects of video information on precolonoscopy anxiety and knowledge: a randomized trial. Lancet. 1999;354(9195):2032–5.
30. Nyman SR, Lucy Y. Usability and acceptability of a website that provides tailored advice on falls prevention activities for older people. Health Informatics J. 2009;15(1):27–39.
31. Herrmann KS, Kreuzer H. A randomized prospective study on anxiety reduction by preparatory disclosure with and without video film show about a planned heart catheterization. Eur Heart J. 1989;10(8):753–7.
32. Spitzer HF. Studies in retention. J Educ Psychol. 1939;30:641–57.

33. Melton AW. The situation with respect to the spacing of repetitions and memory. J Verbal Learn Verbal Behav. 1970;9:596–606.
34. Landauer TK, Bjork RA. Optimum rehearsal patterns and name learning. In: Gruneberg M, Morris PE, Sykes RN, editors. Practical aspects of memory. London: Academic; 1978. p. 625–32.
35. Kirsch IS, Jungeblut A, Jenkins L, Kolstad A. Adult literacy in America: a first look at the results of the National Adult Literacy Survey (NALS). Washington, DC: National Center for Education Statistics, U.S. Department of Education; 1993.
36. Safeer RS, Keenan J. Health literacy: the gap between physicians and patients. Am Fam Physician. 2005;72(3):463–8.
37. Eltorai AE, Sharma P, Wang J, Daniels AH. Most American academy of orthopaedic surgeons' online patient education material exceeds average patient reading level. Clin Orthop Relat Res. 2015;473(4):1181–6.
38. Doak CC, Doak LG, Root JH. Teaching patients with low literacy skills. 2nd ed. Philadelphia: Lippincott; 1996. p. 57–68.
39. Doak CC, Doak LG, Friedell GH, Meade CD. Improving comprehension for cancer patients with low literacy skills: strategies for clinicians. CA Cancer J Clin. 1998;48:151–62.
40. Organization for Economic Co-operation and Development. Time for the US to reskill? What the survey of adult skills says: OECD skills studies. East Jerusalem: OECD Publishing; 2013.
41. US Department of Education, National Center for education statistics. The NAEP Reading achievement levels by grade. Washington, DC: US Department of Education; 2011.
42. Theiss MM, Ellison MW, Tea CG, Warner JF, Silver RM, Murphy VJ. The connection between strong social support and joint replacement outcomes. Orthopedics. 2011;34(5):357.
43. Basques BA, Toy JO, Bohl DD, Golinvaux NS, Grauer JN. General compared with spinal anesthesia for total hip arthroplasty. J Bone Joint Surg Am. 2015;97:455–61.
44. Pugely AJ, Martin CT, Gao Y, Mendoza-Lattes S, Callaghan JJ. Differences in short-term complications between spinal and general anesthesia for primary total knee arthroplasty. J Bone Joint Surg Am. 2013;95:193–9.
45. Macfarlane AJR, Arun Prasad G, Chan VWS, Brull R. Does regional anesthesia improve outcome after total knee arthroplasty? Clin Orthop Relat Res. 2009;467:2379–402.
46. Macfarlane AJR, Prasad GA, Chan VWS, Brull R. Does regional anaesthesia improve outcome after total hip arthroplasty? A systematic review. Br J Anaesth. 2009;103:335–45.
47. Helwani MA, Avidan MS, Ben Abdallah A, Kaiser DJ, Clohisy JC, Hall BL, et al. Effects of regional versus general anesthesia on outcomes after total hip arthroplasty: a retrospective propensity-matched cohort study. J Bone Joint Surg Am. 2015;97:186–93.
48. Stambough JB, Bloom GB, Edwards PK, Mehaffey GR, Barnes CL, Mears SC. Rapid recovery after total joint arthroplasty using general anesthesia. J Arthroplast. 2019;34(9):1889–96.
49. Kee JR, Edwards PK, Barnes CL, Foster SE, Mears SC. After-hours calls in a joint replacement practice. J Arthroplast. 2019;34:1303–6.

Chapter 17
Outcome Metrics: What to Measure Now and in the Future

Robert Pivec and Jess H. Lonner

Introduction

Recognition that total joint arthroplasty (TJA) represents the highest single expenditure for the Centers for Medicare and Medicaid Services (CMS) has been a catalyst for the implementation of alternative treatment and cost containment initiatives for total hip and knee replacement, irrespective of payer [1]. Interest in outpatient TJA has paralleled changes at the Federal level, particularly with a shift towards Alternative Payment Models (APMs), such as the mandatory Comprehensive Care for Joint Replacement (CJR) model started in 2016 or the voluntary Bundled Payments for Care Improvement (BPCI) Advanced model [2]. Furthermore, there is a growing use of ambulatory surgery centers (ASCs) for outpatient TJA in appropriately indicated patients [3, 4]. These broad shifts in both the method of healthcare delivery (outpatient TJA) and the method of reimbursement (APMs) make it incumbent on the surgeon to know which clinical and nonclinical data is collected and tracked. Outcome metrics can be extremely helpful for informing decisions regarding patient selection, protocol development, surgical techniques, site of care, and appropriateness of outpatient TJA. Equally, if not more important, outcomes assessment is critical to ensure that the shift to outpatient TJA does not increase readmissions or complications and that indirect costs are not increased as a result.

R. Pivec · J. H. Lonner (✉)
Rothman Orthopaedic Institute, Philadelphia, PA, USA

Department of Orthopaedic Surgery, Sidney Kimmel Medical College of Thomas Jefferson University, Philadelphia, PA, USA
e-mail: Robert.Pivec@RothmanOrtho.com; Jess.Lonner@RothmanOrtho.com

R. M. Meneghini, L. T. Buller (eds.), *Outpatient Hip and Knee Replacement*,
https://doi.org/10.1007/978-3-031-27037-6_17

Assessing Success: Patient-Report Outcomes and Satisfaction Scores

Patient-reported outcome measures (PROMs) are the foundation of assessing clinical outcomes following TJA. Although there are numerous PROMs to choose from, the authors routinely obtain Lower Extremity Function (LEF), Knee Injury and Osteoarthritis Outcome Score (KOOS)/Hip Disability and Osteoarthritis Outcome Score (HOOS), 12-Item Short Form Mental and Physical Component Survey (SF-12 MCS and PCS), and New Knee Society Scores both at the initial visit and at subsequent follow-up visits. These outcome metrics represent both disease-specific and general health scores and have historically been utilized primarily for research purposes. More recently, some of these have been used by payers to quantify the quality of care and determine value-based payments. It is anticipated that value-based care payment initiatives will increasingly rely on PROMs to influence compensation for care. Collection of PROMs enables the surgeon and care team to monitor their own TJA patient outcomes longitudinally. Common validated outcome measures such as KOOS, HOOS, Oxford Knee Scores, and New Knee Society Scoring systems are useful surgery-specific tools for knee and hip arthroplasty [5, 6].

The utility of disease-specific PROMs such as Western Ontario and McMaster University Osteoarthritis Index (WOMAC), Oxford Hip Score, and Knee Society Clinical Rating Score (KSCRS) was demonstrated by Halawi et al. to have a higher correlation with patient satisfaction than general health scores (e.g., SF-12), activity (e.g., UCLA Activity Score), or perceptions of normalcy [5]. More specifically, the authors observed that of disease-specific PROMs, the pain domain was most closely correlated with patient satisfaction [4].

Patient satisfaction is increasingly recognized as an important measure of outcome after TJA, which was often ignored in classic PROMs. Patient satisfaction with ASC care is collected through a CMS program termed Consumer Assessment of Healthcare Providers and Systems Outpatient and Ambulatory Surgery Survey (OAS CAHPS), which mirrors the inpatient side of hospital satisfaction reporting (HCAHPS). However, unlike its inpatient cousin, OAS CAHPS is a voluntary program started by CMS in 2016. As of 2022, it remains a voluntary initiative per CMS. Although ASCs at this time are not monetarily penalized for low satisfaction scores (unlike inpatient procedures which are monitored via HCAHPS), this type of revenue-penalty model, which has been termed Value-Based Purchasing (VBP) by CMS, was mandated to be implemented for ASCs as well by the Affordable Care Act (ACA).

Pain management has been well-documented to impact satisfaction scores; therefore, surgeons should collect metrics that include patient satisfaction, particularly since it is tied to HCAHPS (and likely OAS CAHPS in the future) and hospital reimbursement via the VBP program. Prior studies have demonstrated that low HCAHPS scores were primarily correlated with poor pain control, which led to increased emphasis on pain management. Thus, the measurement of patient satisfaction, as it relates to pain management, will become increasingly important in the future as VBP programs transition from the inpatient side to ASCs. In a recent study assessing the correlation between pain and low patient satisfaction scores, Jung et al. demonstrated that patient satisfaction was actually better correlated with a shorter length-of-stay (LOS) than pain [7]. Data is now emerging showing that the inherently shorter LOSs with ASCs are translating into higher patient satisfaction compared to inpatient TJA. A recent study by Kelly et al. demonstrated that compared to inpatient surgery, outpatient TJA patients were more satisfied—particularly with regards to pain management, nurse responsiveness, and thoroughness of discharge planning—and preferred the outpatient procedures [8].

While we do not expect any clinically meaningful changes in longer term joint-specific outcomes measures when TJA surgeries are transitioned to the outpatient setting, cost of care and patient satisfaction may be improved. Additionally, attention to outcomes metrics should assist the surgeon and institution in informing patient selection and perioperative protocols, mitigating risk, controlling costs, and improving outcomes in outpatient TJA. The onus is on us to ensure that the shift to outpatient care does not increase readmissions, complications, or indirect costs, and it is our responsibility to carefully track these particular outcomes with regards to outpatient TJA.

Assessing Safety: Complications

It is recommended that surgeons routinely track their complications and need for hospital readmissions, ensuring that they are not occurring with greater frequency in the outpatient compared to the inpatient settings. Healy et al. and Iorio et al. have published comprehensive standardized lists of complications of both TKA and THA that may serve as useful resources (Table 17.1) [9–11].

Complications are recorded, tracked, and publicly reported by CMS. For the inpatient setting, there are currently eight complications with mandated reporting and public disclosure (Table 17.2). The complications are then compared to other hospitals in the local region to identify statistical outliers (defined as outside of the 95% confidence interval bounds for the region) and publicly reported on a per-hospital basis using a color-coded scheme (Table 17.3).

Similar reporting models apply to ASCs, where reimbursement is tied to compliance with CMS reporting requirements, including provisions for public reporting, via the Ambulatory Surgical Center Quality Reporting Program (ASCQR). If ASCs do not comply with reporting requirements, they may incur a 2% reduction to any future ASC Medicare payment update thereby decreasing revenues. Although not TJA-specific, some of these complications do pertain to hip and knee replacement including wrong site surgery, patient falls, and transfers to acute care hospitals (Table 17.4). Certainly, the latter two risks are of great concern in the outpatient setting and may be mitigated with careful patient selection and meticulous perioperative management.

Table 17.1 Complications for knee and hip arthroplasty as defined by the Knee Society [9] and Hip Society [11]

Complications for total knee arthroplasty	Complications for total hip arthroplasty
1. Bleeding	1. Bleeding
2. Wound complication	2. Wound complication
3. Thromboembolic disease	3. Thromboembolic disease
4. Neural deficit	4. Neural deficit
5. Vascular injury	5. Vascular injury
6. Medial collateral ligament injury	6. Dislocation/instability
7. Instability	7. Periprosthetic fracture
8. Malalignment	8. Abductor muscle disruption
9. Stiffness	9. Deep periprosthetic joint infection
10. Deep periprosthetic joint infection	10. Heterotopic ossification
11. Periprosthetic fracture	11. Bearing surface wear
12. Extensor mechanism disruption	12. Osteolysis
13. Patellofemoral dislocation	13. Implant loosening
14. Tibiofemoral dislocation	14. Cup-liner dissociation
15. Bearing surface wear	15. Implant fracture
16. Osteolysis	16. Reoperation
17. Implant loosening	17. Revision
18. Implant fracture or tibial insert dissociation	18. Readmission
19. Reoperation	19. Death
20. Revision	
21. Readmission	
22. Death	

Table 17.2 Complications tracked and reported by CMS

Complication	Reporting period
Acute myocardial infarction (AMI)	7 days of admission
Pneumonia	7 days of admission
Sepsis/septic shock	7 days of admission
Surgical site bleeding	30 days of admission
Pulmonary embolism	30 days of admission
Death	30 days of admission
Mechanical complications	90 days of admission
Periprosthetic joint infection/wound infection	90 days of admission

Assessing Failure: Readmissions

Readmissions or transfers following outpatient TJA, if performed in the outpatient hospital setting, or transfers/admission to the hospital from the ASC setting, are both tracked and publicly reported by CMS. Again, these occurrences, regardless of payer, should be closely followed by surgeons in order to maintain a high level of patient care and ideally should be reviewed on a month-by-month basis to ensure that patient selection and perioperative protocols are acceptable [12].

Table 17.3 CMS reporting criteria for complications

Category	Better than the national rate	No different than the national rate	Worse than the national rate	The number of cases is too small
Criterion	The entire 95% interval estimate surrounding the hospital's rate is lower than the national rate	The 95% interval estimate surrounding the hospital's rate includes the national rate	The entire 95% interval estimate surrounding the hospital's rate is higher than the national rate	Fewer than 25 cases

Table 17.4 Ambulatory surgery center reporting mandates pertaining to TJA

Reporting Code	Complication
ASC-1	Patient burn
ASC-2	Patient fall
ASC-3	Wrong site, wrong side, wrong patient, wrong procedure, wrong implant
ASC-4	All-cause hospital transfer/admission
ASC-13	Normothermia

CMS tracks six procedures (including hip and knee replacement) and levies a penalty if the readmission rate is above a certain threshold, except for exempt institutions (such as VA, rural hospitals, Children's hospitals, among others) [13]. If TJA is performed in a hospital outpatient setting, the institution may be liable for readmissions for a maximum penalty of 3% Medicare revenue per year under the Hospital Readmissions Reduction Program (HRRP). [13, 14] A recent study by Springer et al. demonstrated a higher readmission rate for outpatient TJA (11.7%) compared to inpatient TJA (6.6%). Many of these readmissions were either due to poor pain control at home or wound complications. Interestingly, despite higher readmission rates, patients who underwent outpatient TJA were significantly more satisfied than inpatients [15].

On the ambulatory side, CMS tracks the number of patients that require transfer/admission to a hospital from an ASC (Table 17.4). Another proposed rule in 2019 has evaluated the possibility of adding a further tracked metric for Emergency Department (ED) visits and admissions within 7 days of various ASC procedures, including TJA. However, at this time the proposed rule is limited to General Surgery procedures only, for tracked diagnoses such as bleeding or DVT/PE. Currently, no financial penalties have been levied (CMS currently only requires compliance with reporting outcomes via the ASCQR program). However, it is possible that revenue may be withheld with future CMS rule changes if ASC transfer and/or admission rates are above a certain threshold, similar to the HRRP. While CMS has formalized some of these policies, and though CMS-insured patients are not the common demographic for outpatient TJA, private payers often follow the lead of CMS and may eventually impose similar penalties for admissions.

While there is some incentive for surgeon practices with bundled payment arrangements with private insurances and CMS to transition TJA to an outpatient setting in ASCs, complications and hospital admissions or transfers can have a large financial impact given the practices' assumed risk for costs for the entire episode of care. Surgeons will need to keep a close eye on both their readmission rates, but also their transfer and post-discharge ED visits particularly if performing outpatient TJA in an ASC. Better screening of patients preoperatively to optimize patients and appropriately select patients for the outpatient setting, optimized perioperative management protocols, as well as perioperative navigation and access to the care team, may help decrease complications, unnecessary ED visits, and readmission rates [16].

Assessing Costs: Healthcare Costs in the CJR Era

Across a broad spectrum of procedures, Medicare estimated savings of almost $7 billion between 2007 through 2011 and up to $12 billion between 2012 through 2017 by shifting outpatient surgical procedures from hospitals to ASCs for patients considered low-risk [17]. While the typical targeted demographic for outpatient TJA is not necessarily the Medicare-aged population, but rather the younger patient cohort, the general message is the same. Payers may stand to save a great deal of money if carefully selected TJA cases are transitioned to the ASC. In APM and bundled care arrangements, hospitals and physicians may be held accountable for costs for an entire 90-day episode of care and are required to pay a penalty if spending following TJA exceeds what is termed the quality-adjusted spending benchmark [18, 19]. Although the CJR model was designed in an era of inpatient TJA, in the future surgeons need to be prepared for ongoing CMS rule changes, and shifting models of reimbursement by private payers, to align reimbursement models between inpatient and outpatient procedures. [20]

Surgeons also need to be aware of the difference in reimbursement for TJA in the inpatient versus ambulatory setting, which can range anywhere from 18 to 28% less if performed in an outpatient setting. One further layer of added complexity is differentiating between the hospital outpatient department (HOPD) and an ASC which also have further reimbursement differentials, with similar procedures performed in an ASC reimbursed at rates ~20% lower than if done in a HOPD [18, 19]. In many non-Medicare bundled care arrangements, total costs per episode of care after total and partial joint arthroplasty may also prove a beneficial cost impact from transitioning to outpatient cases, as long as complications and indirect costs are mitigated during the episode of care.

The ability to accurately measure costs will be paramount for efficient operation in the ambulatory setting. A recent study by Palsis et al. evaluated two different methods of accounting for TJA: traditional accounting and what is termed time-driven activity-based costing (TDABC) [20]. The authors noted that while fixed costs such as implant costs or surgeon's fees were accurately accounted for with traditional accounting, indirect costs and space/equipment costs were substantially overestimated with traditional account methods. The authors concluded that for total knee arthroplasty traditional accounting produced a negative margin of 36%, when CMS payments were used as a revenue source, and a positive margin of 22% when TDABC methods were used. Thus, it is critical that surgeons, particularly those with ownership or gain-sharing arrangements with ASCs ensure they have a robust accounting capability that accurately manages the costs of care.

Conclusion

Outcomes metrics is a term that represents a vast array of potential data that can be collected and analyzed for patients undergoing TJA. Although there is some overlap, outcomes metrics that are of primary interest to the surgeon to help inform and guide improvements in perioperative surgical care may not align with the metrics that are preferred by regulatory agencies such as CMS or commercial insurance providers. Surgeons may find it informative, effective, and efficient to adopt systems to effectively track useful outcomes measures while remaining in compliance with regulatory bodies for patient data reporting. In the case of outpatient knee and hip arthroplasty, the key outcomes measures to assess are costs of care, patient satisfaction, and the risks of complications, Emergency Department visits, and hospital transfers/admissions. While functional outcomes measures will likely not show obvious differences when surgery is performed on an outpatient or inpatient basis, our responsibility is to confirm that we can deliver outpatient TJA safely and cost-effectively in the outpatient setting, and that patients are equally, if not more satisfied compared to those receiving inpatient TJA. These are important outcomes measures for us to track longitudinally and frequently, as we work to refine indications for outpatient surgery, inform patient selection criteria, influence perioperative protocols for patient care and access to the care team, and expand the numbers of knee and hip replacements performed in ASCs.

References

1. Kim H, Meath THA, Dobbertin K, Quiñones AR, Ibrahim SA, Mcconnell KJ. Association of the mandatory medicare bundled payment with joint replacement outcomes in hospitals with disadvantaged patients. JAMA Netw Open. 2019;2(11):1–13. https://doi.org/10.1001/jamanetworkopen.2019.14696.
2. Manickas-Hill O, Feeley T, Bozic KJ. A review of bundled payments in total joint replacement. JBJS Rev. 2019;7(11):e1. https://doi.org/10.2106/JBJS.RVW.18.00169.
3. Parcells BW, Giacobbe D, Macknet D, et al. Total joint arthroplasty in a stand-alone ambulatory surgical center: short-term outcomes. Orthopedics. 2016;39(4):223–8. https://doi.org/10.3928/01477447-20160419-06.
4. Shah RR, Cipparrone NE, Gordon AC, Raab DJ, Bresch JR, Shah NA. Is it safe? Outpatient total joint arthroplasty with discharge to home at a freestanding ambulatory surgical center. Arthroplast Today. 2018;4(4):484–7. https://doi.org/10.1016/j.artd.2018.08.002.

5. Halawi MJ, Jongbloed W, Baron S, Savoy L, Cote MP, Lieberman JR. Patient-reported outcome measures are not a valid proxy for patient satisfaction in total joint arthroplasty. J Arthroplast. 2019;35:3–7. https://doi.org/10.1016/j.arth.2019.09.033.
6. Scuderi GR, Bourne RB, Noble PC, Benjamin JB, Lonner JH, Scott WN. The new knee society knee scoring system. Clin Orthop Relat Res. 2012;470(1):3–19. https://doi.org/10.1007/s11999-011-2135-0.
7. Jung EK, Srivastava K, Abouljoud M, Keller R, Okoroha K, Davis J. Does hospital consumer assessment of healthcare providers and systems survey correlate with traditional metrics of patient satisfaction? The challenge of measuring patient pain control and satisfaction in total joint replacement. Arthroplast Today. 2018;4(4):470–4. https://doi.org/10.1016/j.artd.2018.02.009.
8. Kelly MP, Calkins TE, Culvern C, Kogan M, Della Valle CJ. Inpatient versus outpatient hip and knee arthroplasty: which has higher patient satisfaction? J Arthroplast. 2018;33(11):3402–6. https://doi.org/10.1016/j.arth.2018.07.025.
9. Healy WL, Della Valle CJ, Iorio R, et al. Complications of total knee arthroplasty: standardized list and definitions of the knee society. Clin Orthop Relat Res. 2013;471(1):215–20. https://doi.org/10.1007/s11999-012-2489-y.
10. Iorio R, Della Valle CJ, Healy WL, et al. Stratification of standardized TKA complications and adverse events: a brief communication. Clin Orthop Relat Res. 2014;472(1):194–205. https://doi.org/10.1007/s11999-013-2980-0.
11. Healy WL, Iorio R, Clair AJ, Pellegrini VD, Della Valle CJ, Berend KR. Complications of total hip arthroplasty: standardized list, definitions, and stratification developed by the hip society. Clin Orthop Relat Res. 2016;474(2):357–64. https://doi.org/10.1007/s11999-015-4341-7.
12. Public Policy Institute A. Insight on the issues impact of the medicare hospital readmission reduction program on hospital readmissions following joint replacement surgery. 2015.
13. Li BY, Urish KL, Jacobs BL, et al. Inaugural readmission penalties for total hip and total knee arthroplasty procedures under the hospital readmissions reduction program. JAMA Netw Open. 2019;2(11):e1916008. https://doi.org/10.1001/jamanetworkopen.2019.16008.
14. Cassard X, Garnault V, Corin B, Claverie D, Murgier J. Outpatient total knee arthroplasty: readmission and complication rates on day 30 in 61 patients. Orthop Traumatol Surg Res. 2018;104(7):967–70. https://doi.org/10.1016/j.otsr.2018.07.014.
15. Springer BD, Odum SM, Vegari DN, Mokris JG, Beaver WB. Impact of inpatient versus outpatient total joint arthroplasty on 30-day hospital readmission rates and unplanned episodes of care. Orthop Clin North Am. 2017;48(1):15–23. https://doi.org/10.1016/j.ocl.2016.08.002.
16. Ziemba-Davis M, Caccavallo P, Meneghini RM. Outpatient joint arthroplasty—patient selection: update on the outpatient arthroplasty risk assessment score. J Arthroplast. 2019;34(7):S40–3. https://doi.org/10.1016/j.arth.2019.01.007.
17. Levinson DR, General I. Medicare and beneficiaries could save billions if CMS reduces hospital outpatient department payment rates for ambulatory surgical center-approved procedures to ambulatory surgical center payment rates, A-05-12-00020. 2014. https://oig.hhs.gov/oas/reports/region5/51200020.pdf.
18. Piccinin MA, Sayeed Z, Kozlowski R, Bobba V, Knesek D, Frush T. Bundle payment for musculoskeletal care: current evidence (part 1). Orthop Clin North Am. 2018;49(2):135–46. https://doi.org/10.1016/j.ocl.2017.11.002.
19. Piccinin MA, Sayeed Z, Kozlowski R, Bobba V, Knesek D, Frush T. Bundle payment for musculoskeletal care: current evidence (part 2). Orthop Clin North Am. 2018;49(2):147–56. https://doi.org/10.1016/j.ocl.2017.11.003.
20. Palsis JA, Brehmer TS, Pellegrini VD, Drew JM, Sachs BL. The cost of joint replacement comparing two approaches to evaluating costs of total hip and knee arthroplasty. J Bone Jt Surg Am. 2018;100(4):326–33. https://doi.org/10.2106/JBJS.17.00161.

Chapter 18
How to Mitigate Risk for Surgeons, Institutions, and Patients

Leonard T. Buller and R. Michael Meneghini

Introduction

Total joint arthroplasty (TJA) is an excellent treatment for disabling joint disease [1]. Since its original description, the primary goals of TJA have remained constant: to perform a durable reconstruction that reduces pain, restores function, and improves the quality of life [2]. Until recently, multiple days of inpatient care following TJA was the expectation. Lately, there has been a transition from a "sick-patient" to a "well-patient" model, whereby patients are optimized prior to surgery and no longer require prolonged in-hospital care. Simultaneously, refinements in surgical technique, multimodal pain management, blood conservation, and physical therapy have resulted in quicker recovery and a transition to outpatient TJA [3]. Interest in outpatient TJA has also been driven by financial considerations, like surgeon ownership of ambulatory surgery centers (ASCs) [4]. The pressure to transition to outpatient TJA was further escalated in the United States with the Outpatient Prospective Payment System 2018 rule, which removed TKA from the inpatient-only list, causing hospitals and payers to treat all Medicare TKA patients as outpatients [5]. All of these factors provided a groundwork for developing rapid recovery protocols to accommodate early discharge after TJA. However, the safety of outpatient TJA remains a concern. This chapter describes how to minimize risk to patients, surgeons, and institutions through appropriate preoperative evaluation, optimization, and multidisciplinary care coordination.

L. T. Buller (✉) · R. M. Meneghini
Department of Orthopaedic Surgery, Indiana University School of Medicine, Indianapolis, IN, USA
e-mail: mmeneghini@injri.com

R. M. Meneghini, L. T. Buller (eds.), *Outpatient Hip and Knee Replacement*,
https://doi.org/10.1007/978-3-031-27037-6_18

Reducing Patient Risk

Reducing risk in outpatient TJA begins well before the patient enters the operating room; commencing with appropriate surgical indications, as even the best surgery on the wrong patient will yield more harm than benefit. Risk stratification and preoperative optimization, as described in the first two chapters, is mandatory for all patients undergoing elective TJA. The preoperative evaluation should include medical, dental, and where appropriate cardiac clearances, medication reconciliations, and a venous thromboembolism prophylaxis plan [6]. The medical team is responsible for identifying and correcting any modifiable risk factors. Multiple new medical diagnoses are made during prescreening and up to 2.5% of patients are considered to have unacceptably high surgical risk for elective TJA [7]. Furthermore, only a minority of patients lack comorbidities (13% of total knee arthroplasties (TKAs) and 17% of total hip arthroplasties (THAs)), emphasizing the importance of prescreening [8].

After preoperative optimization, selecting those patients appropriate for outpatient TJA has traditionally been limited to nonspecific surrogates such as the American Society of Anesthesiologists Physical Status (ASA-PS) classification or the Charlson Comorbidity Index (CCI), which were not specifically designed for this purpose. Surgeons often combine these indices with the knowledge that certain medical comorbidities are associated with longer hospital stays [9], and select patients without these conditions for an outpatient pathway [10]. However, this selection strategy is not evidence-based and has been shown in multiple studies to result in poor reliability in identifying those patients capable of outpatient TJA [11, 12], underscoring the importance of accurate risk stratification for safe patient selection. This is particularly important when considering most outpatient TJA studies are performed within the safety net of outpatient hospital departments, where patients who do not meet discharge criteria can be converted to an inpatient hospitalization. As the expansion of outpatient TJA in ASCs continues, risk reduction through appropriate patient selection will become critical.

The Outpatient Arthroplasty Risk Assessment (OARA) score was specifically designed to identify patients medically appropriate for same- and next-day discharge after TJA. Appreciating the vulnerabilities of outpatient TJA patients, the OARA score was specifically designed to err in the direction of patient safety and multiple studies have evaluated its validity [13, 14]. Using a preoperative cutoff of 79 points, the OARA score approaches the desired 100% positive predictive value (PPV), 100% specificity, and 0% False Positive Rate (FPR). The high PPV, or probability that patients with lower scores were discharged home the same day, and specificity, or proportion of patients with higher scores who did not go home the same day; combined with the low FPR, or proportion of patients with higher scores who went home the same day, indicates that the OARA score effectively identifies patients who can safely undergo outpatient TJA. Additionally, the low Negative Predictive Value, or probability that patients with a higher score were not discharged the same day, low sensitivity, or proportion of patients with a lower score who were discharged the same day, and high False Negative Rate, or proportion of patients with a lower score who did not go home the same day, reflects the design of the score to err in the direction of patient safety. Accurate risk stratification, using evidence-based selection criteria, is a critical step in reducing patient risk in outpatient TJA.

A patient's fear and anxiety of the unknown and pain is a primary barrier to outpatient TJA [15, 16]. However, there are multiple benefits from recovering in the home environment including elimination of nosocomial risks and institutional disturbances, as well as access to preferred foods and leisure objects. Expectation setting through a unified, team-based approach is crucial in alleviating patient fears and explaining the benefits of outpatient TJA. Preoperative patient education begins in the office at the initial visit with written and electronic patient educational materials. Standardized patient education positively impacts patient satisfaction, particularly with regard to pain management, which is a leading barrier to early discharge [17]. Additionally, preoperative education improves postoperative outcomes, lowers costs, and reduces lengths of stay [18]. Expectations for recovery should be communicated to patients in all educational materials and by all staff involved in patient care. The expectations should include a discussion of the disease process and entire phase of care, the location of recovery and/or therapy, pain expectations, ambulation expectations, driving expectations, and return to work expectations. More information is covered in a shorter period of time and an emphasis should be placed on how to manage variability in pain, nausea, swelling, and other symptoms that the patients may experience for the first time at home. Appropriate optimization, risk stratification, and preoperative education are all strategies that reduce patient risk. However, surgeon and institution variables are also responsible for reducing patient risk in outpatient TJA.

Reducing Surgeon Risk

Appropriate surgical indication for TJA is the first way to reduce surgeon risk. Surgeons should assure the patient's specific disease pattern makes them likely to benefit from outpatient TJA. This includes utilizing tools that predict patients at risk of a poor outcome [19], as well as tools that identify patients at risk for failure of early discharge [20]. While outpatient TJA results in less rounding, lower inpatient burden, and fewer healthcare provider "touches," the overall patient care commitment is not less [21], including an increase in the number of phone calls [22]. The shift in perioperative care burden from the hospital to caregivers [23] and the surgical team mandates enhancement of outpatient staff accessibility [24]. Multiple strategies exist to increase staff availability including hiring more staff, extending clinic hours, scheduling preemptive telephone calls, or utilizing technologies to monitor patient recovery [25, 26]. A safety net is required to assure patient well-being, minimize complications, and reduce readmissions. When patients are discharged home earlier, they are more isolated and oftentimes geographically distanced from their surgeon. Regardless of discharge disposition and timing, postsurgical patients still have the same risks of complications after surgery. Therefore, a successful outpatient TJA must include a safety net to minimize the risk of feeling or experiencing abandonment.

Surgeon risk can also be reduced by understanding how a predictable set of complications routinely delays patient discharge in an outpatient pathway: blood pressure (hypotension or hypertension), over-sedation, postoperative urinary retention (POUR), postoperative nausea and/or vomiting, pain and social support issues [27]. To reduce surgeon risk, each of these should be considered in detail before outpatient TJA. Additionally, establishing a way to track and monitor outcomes is critical to assess the strengths and weaknesses of individual protocols. These protocols can then be modified based on this data, further reducing surgeon risk. Important protocols to develop during the establishment of an outpatient TJA pathway include pain management (multimodal drugs and narcotic minimization), anesthesia, blood and fluid management, and surgical technique. Though previously discussed in other chapters, we will briefly address each of these and their role in reducing surgeon risk.

Multimodal pain management, through an established pathway, in combination with technically excellent surgery and anesthesia that reduces side effects and complications is crucial to expediting recovery. The goals are to minimize pain, sedation, hypoventilation, urinary retention, and nausea while encouraging early mobilization. A multimodal approach that starts before surgery and includes protocols after the patient is discharged home has been demonstrated by many high-volume centers to result in successful rapid recovery after TJA [28–33].

The choice of anesthesia varies by surgeon and anesthesiologist preference, but the two teams should cooperate with the mutual understanding of the goal of early mobilization. Anesthesia should provide adequate sedation and pain control intraoperatively, as well as maintain a level of postoperative pain control while minimizing confusion, sedation, and nausea. Neuraxial anesthesia decreases postoperative narcotic use, decreases cardiopulmonary morbidity, decreases the risk of thromboembolic events, decreases blood loss, and optimizes muscle relaxation, which eases surgical exposure [34–36]. When done correctly, a short-acting spinal with a half-life of 2 h provides an early motor return, allowing for participation in physical therapy shortly after completion of the procedure. Regional anesthesia is also helpful in postoperative pain management, decreasing the need for narcotics, allowing earlier ambulation, and reducing the rate of readmissions and hospital length of stay [37–40]. Soft tissue, peri- and intra-articular injections have also been demonstrated, in multiple administration forms, to reduce postoperative pain, decrease the need for oral narcotics, and improve range of motion [41–43].

Attention to blood and fluid management is critical, as blood loss remains a concern for the safety of outpatient TJA; particularly in ASCs, where blood transfusions are often unavailable. Development of an effective blood management strategy begins with identifying patients who may be at risk for requiring postoperative transfusion [44, 45] and incorporating modern transfusion protocols that include both the hemoglobin level as well as patient symptoms. The widespread use of tranexamic acid has dramatically reduced perioperative blood loss and transfusions

[46, 47], without increasing thromboembolic complications [48], and should be given to all eligible patients [49–51].

Perioperative hydration is also crucial to reduce the number of postoperative complications that prevent outpatient TJA, including POUR. The American Society of Anesthesiologists guidelines should be utilized, which encourages patients who meet the appropriate criteria to drink clear liquids up to 2 h before surgery [52]. Intraoperative IV hydration ensures intravascular volumes are sufficient to minimize orthostatic hypotension, tachycardia, and low urine output. Rapid recovery protocols should aim for approximately two liters of intraoperative IV crystalloids, with an additional 1 L postoperatively. Despite a low relative incidence, the use of rocuronium, glycopyrrolate, neostigmine, and fentanyl spinals are associated with POUR and their use in the perioperative period should be minimized [53].

Finally, the influence of surgical approach on the ability to undergo outpatient TJA should be considered in as much as the surgeon should be comfortable with the chosen approach and must be diligent to minimize intraoperative complications. When effectively executed, surgical approach does not appear to have a significant influence on overall postoperative pain, length of stay, or ability to mobilize [54]. The focus should be on maximizing efficiency and streamlining the procedure, removing extraneous steps or delays and minimizing complications. Surgeons and teams should be aware that introducing new techniques is associated with a learning curve, which may result in increased blood loss, complications, and time [55]. Operating room efficiency is the key and surgeons should surround themselves with staff who make the procedure run as smoothly as possible. Everyone involved should know their steps to limit errors and reduce risk.

Reducing Institution Risk

After appropriate patient selection and optimization, a multidisciplinary approach to outpatient TJA is critical to assure the procedure is performed safely and with a low risk of complications. The first step in reducing institutional risk is convincing institution administration that their support of an outpatient TJA pathway will be directly beneficial by improving bed availability and reducing exposure to expenses [56]. Hospital and ASC insurance contracting is crucial to assure the insurance pre-approval process identifies facility-fee reimbursement issues and non-covered patient costs. Some insurers consider TJA performed at an ASC "out of network." Therefore, it is critical to obtain credentialing for outpatient TJA and do a thorough pro forma based on the payer mix, meet with the payers, and negotiate rates for each procedure. With regards to Medicare patients, many hospitals are charged early discharge penalties for outpatient TJA and identifying these situations ahead of time can minimize the financial burden on the patient and should be a part of the institutional screening program for outpatient TJA.

A multidisciplinary approach to outpatient TJA dramatically reduces lengths of stay and readmission rates, while enabling earlier ambulation [29]. We recommend creating a routine coordinated care conference attended by key members of the multidisciplinary team to discuss upcoming surgeries. The goal of this meeting is to share information across disciplines, anticipate and answer questions, and proactively develop patient care plans. The team members should include the surgeon, anesthesiologist, hospitalist [57], nursing staff [58], physical therapy, and pharmacy. To further reduce institution risk, as a part of preoperative optimization, specific protocols should be established by the multidisciplinary team to address common medical conditions. For example, smokers should be counseled regarding preoperative cessation to optimize wound healing and reduce anesthesia-related risks. Obese patients should be educated on the increased risks associated with obesity and weight loss recommendations should be established. Similarly, patients with poorly managed diabetes mellitus, a known risk factor for higher postoperative complications [59], should have their procedure delayed until strict glycemic control is attained. Individualized risk stratification for deep vein thromboembolism should also be included [6], and plans for prophylaxis should be made preemptively to avoid delays, confusion, and the risk of readmissions in the postoperative period.

Appropriately selecting patients eligible for outpatient TJA will reduce institutional risk. Unlike ASA-PS and the CCI scores, the OARA score is not a measure of physical status, medical complexity, or mortality but still accounts for comorbid conditions relevant to TJA. This is helpful because some patients who are poor candidates for early discharge may have low ASA-PS and CCI scores. For instance, a patient with a history of poor pain control due to fibromyalgia, who is otherwise healthy, would have an ASA-PS score of 1, and a low CCI but a high OARA score, making them unacceptable for early discharge. In contrast, a patient with multiple but stable medical problems may have higher ASA-PS and CCI scores, but a lower OARA score. Thus, the OARA score helps reduce the institutional risk of inpatient conversions or readmissions through appropriate stratification.

As opposed to being with similar patients in the inpatient setting, recovery within an outpatient protocol is more likely to occur in isolation. Consequently, the importance of a "Joint class" or "Joint camp," in which a group of patients attends a meeting to hear the full details of the procedure, expands patient education beyond didactic materials. This allows patients to socialize and work together through questions and answers. Joint classes have been demonstrated to decrease lengths of stay by nearly 50% and increase the likelihood of timely discharge by 62% [60]. Standardized reading material in these classes is useful as a reference to answer patient questions, but the institution must assure staffing is available to answer specific questions not covered in the handouts.

A final area for risk reduction at the institution level is in the immediate postoperative setting. The goals of immediate postoperative management in outpatient TJA are minimization of pain and early mobilization. During the acute phase, experienced anesthesia and nursing staff transfer the patient from the operating room to the post-anesthesia care unit to stabilize them medically and manage pain and nausea. During the step-down phase, patients are transferred to a private recovery area where they begin rehabilitation and are educated on proper wound care and how to assess for signs of complications. The institution should assure staff familiar with rapid recovery protocols are available to facilitate this process, which decreases patient anxiety and fear [28, 61]. Finally, a member of the team should be responsible for reaching out to the patient within 24–48 h postoperatively to assess their progress and answer questions.

At the institution level, anticipatory management is advisable to establish and adhere to vetted protocols, as opposed to reacting after a complication or readmission occurs. The importance of data collection to track volume, outcomes, and patient progress cannot be overstated and will assure necessary staff and service line resources are available. While careful patient selection is critical to minimize risk, so is facility and staff selection to maximize operating room efficiency and safety. This includes training staff on patient setup and room layout to facilitate efficient surgery and faster turnover, as well as standardization of instrument trays to reduce setup time and decrease the cost of sterilizing unused instruments. Establishing institutional protocols will decrease risk by improving reproducibility, decreasing operating room times, decreasing time to onboard staff, improving staff confidence, and increasing a surgeon's confidence in their staff.

Conclusion

With increasing pressure to improve efficiency and reduce cost, improvements in our understanding of postoperative recovery have allowed for an evidence-based shift towards outpatient TJA. Rapid recovery TJA has been successfully performed in multiple patient populations, with low rates of complications and readmissions [62, 63], even in elderly patients [64–69]. In its current state, appropriately performed outpatient TJA is a safe [70–73], cost-efficient [4, 74, 75], and patient-friendly strategy [76]. It is projected that greater than half of all primary TJAs will be performed in an outpatient setting by 2026 [77]. Most patients recover in a predictable fashion following surgery [30, 64, 78–81] and standardizing care will increase efficiency and the reproducibility of outcomes. Safe and successful outpatient TJA relies on a number of important factors including patient selection, multidisciplinary care coordination, standardized perioperative protocols, and postoperative management. As the proportion of outpatient TJAs increases, it is crucial to create evidence-based safeguards to minimize patient, surgeon, and institution risk.

References

1. Learmonth ID, Young C, Rorabeck C. The operation of the century: total hip replacement. Lancet. 2007;370(9597):1508–19.
2. Charnley J. Arthroplasty of the hip: a new operation. Lancet. 1961;277(7187):1129–32. https://linkinghub.elsevier.com/retrieve/pii/S0140673661920633.

3. Argenson J-NA, Husted H, Lombardi A, Booth RE, Thienpont E. Global forum: an international perspective on outpatient surgical procedures for adult hip and knee reconstruction. J Bone Joint Surg Am. 2016;98(13):e55. http://www.ncbi.nlm.nih.gov/pubmed/27385689.
4. Aynardi M, Post Z, Ong A, Orozco F, Sukin DC. Outpatient surgery as a means of cost reduction in total hip arthroplasty: a case-control study. HSS J. 2014;10(3):252–5. http://www.ncbi.nlm.nih.gov/pubmed/25264442.
5. Yates AJ, Kerr JM, Froimson MI, Della Valle CJ, Huddleston JI. The unintended impact of the removal of total knee arthroplasty from the center for medicare and medicaid services inpatient-only list. J Arthroplast. 2018;33(12):3602–6. http://www.ncbi.nlm.nih.gov/pubmed/30318252.
6. Lieberman JR, Heckmann N. Venous thromboembolism prophylaxis in total hip arthroplasty and total knee arthroplasty patients. J Am Acad Orthop Surg. 2017;25(12):789–98. http://insights.ovid.com/crossref?an=00124635-201712000-00001.
7. Meding JB, Klay M, Healy A, Ritter MA, Keating EM, Berend ME. The prescreening history and physical in elective total joint arthroplasty. J Arthroplast. 2007;22(6):21–3. http://www.ncbi.nlm.nih.gov/pubmed/17823009.
8. Callaghan JJ, Pugely A, Liu S, Noiseux N, Willenborg M, Peck D. Measuring rapid recovery program outcomes: are all patients candidates for rapid recovery. J Arthroplast. 2015;30(4):531–2. http://www.ncbi.nlm.nih.gov/pubmed/25702594.
9. Courtney PM, Rozell JC, Melnic CM, Lee GC. Who should not undergo short stay hip and knee arthroplasty? Risk factors associated with major medical complications following primary total joint arthroplasty. J Arthroplast. 2015;30(9):1–4. http://www.ncbi.nlm.nih.gov/pubmed/26105617.
10. Lovald S, Ong K, Lau E, Joshi G, Kurtz S, Malkani A. Patient selection in outpatient and short-stay total knee arthroplasty. J Surg Orthop Adv. 2014;23(1):2–8. http://www.ncbi.nlm.nih.gov/pubmed/24641891.
11. Goyal N, Chen AF, Padgett SE, Tan TL, Kheir MM, Hopper RH, et al. Otto Aufranc award: a multicenter, randomized study of outpatient versus inpatient total hip arthroplasty. Clin Orthop Relat Res. 2017;475(2):364–72. http://www.ncbi.nlm.nih.gov/pubmed/27287858
12. Gromov K, Kjærsgaard-Andersen P, Revald P, Kehlet H, Husted H. Feasibility of outpatient total hip and knee arthroplasty in unselected patients. Acta Orthop. 2017;88(5):516–21. http://www.ncbi.nlm.nih.gov/pubmed/28426262.
13. Meneghini RM, Ziemba-Davis M, Ishmael MK, Kuzma AL, Caccavallo P. Safe selection of outpatient joint arthroplasty patients with medical risk stratification: the "outpatient arthroplasty risk assessment score". J Arthroplast. 2017;32(8):2325–31. http://www.ncbi.nlm.nih.gov/pubmed/28390881.
14. Ziemba-Davis M, Caccavallo P, Meneghini RM. Outpatient joint arthroplasty—patient selection: update on the outpatient arthroplasty risk assessment score. J Arthroplast. 2019;34(7):S40–3. http://www.ncbi.nlm.nih.gov/pubmed/30738619.
15. Berend ME, Lackey WG, Carter JL. Outpatient-focused joint arthroplasty is the future: the midwest center for joint replacement experience. J Arthroplast. 2018;33(6):1647–8. http://www.ncbi.nlm.nih.gov/pubmed/29548618.
16. Meneghini RM, Ziemba-Davis M. Patient perceptions regarding outpatient hip and knee arthroplasties. J Arthroplast. 2017;32(9):2701–2705.e1. http://www.ncbi.nlm.nih.gov/pubmed/28527684.
17. Majid N, Lee S, Plummer V. The effectiveness of orthopedic patient education in improving patient outcomes: a systematic review protocol. JBI Database System Rev Implement Rep. 2015;13(1):122–33. http://www.ncbi.nlm.nih.gov/pubmed/26447013.
18. Moyer R, Ikert K, Long K, Marsh J. The value of preoperative exercise and education for patients undergoing total hip and knee arthroplasty. JBJS Rev. 2017;5(12):e2. http://www.ncbi.nlm.nih.gov/pubmed/29232265.

19. Twiggs JG, Wakelin EA, Fritsch BA, Liu DW, Solomon MI, Parker DA, et al. Clinical and statistical validation of a probabilistic prediction tool of total knee arthroplasty outcome. J Arthroplast. 2019;34(11):2624–31. http://www.ncbi.nlm.nih.gov/pubmed/31262622.
20. Kim KY, Feng JE, Anoushiravani AA, Dranoff E, Davidovitch RI, Schwarzkopf R. Rapid discharge in total hip arthroplasty: utility of the outpatient arthroplasty risk assessment tool in predicting same-day and next-day discharge. J Arthroplast. 2018;33(8):2412–6. http://www.ncbi.nlm.nih.gov/pubmed/29656963.
21. Shah RP, Karas V, Berger RA. Rapid discharge and outpatient total joint arthroplasty introduce a burden of care to the surgeon. J Arthroplast. 2019;34(7):1307–11. http://www.ncbi.nlm.nih.gov/pubmed/31031153.
22. Sah A. Considerations for office and staff protocols for outpatient joint replacement. J Arthroplast. 2019;34(7):S44–5. https://www.sciencedirect.com/science/article/pii/S0883540319300087.
23. Manohar A, Cheung K, Wu CL, Stierer TS. Burden incurred by patients and their caregivers after outpatient surgery: a prospective observational study. Clin Orthop Relat Res. 2014;472(5):1416–26. http://link.springer.com/10.1007/s11999-013-3270-6.
24. Billon L, Décaudin B, Pasquier G, Lons A, Deken-Delannoy V, Germe A-F, et al. Prospective assessment of patients' knowledge and informational needs and of surgeon-to-patient information transfer before and after knee or hip arthroplasty. Orthop Traumatol Surg Res. 2017;103(8):1161–7. http://www.ncbi.nlm.nih.gov/pubmed/28964919.
25. Hällfors E, Saku SA, Mäkinen TJ, Madanat R. A consultation phone service for patients with total joint arthroplasty may reduce unnecessary emergency department visits. J Arthroplast. 2018;33(3):650–4. http://www.ncbi.nlm.nih.gov/pubmed/29157787.
26. Jayakumar P, Di J, Fu J, Craig J, Joughin V, Nadarajah V, et al. A patient-focused technology-enabled program improves outcomes in primary total hip and knee replacement surgery. JBJS Open Access. 2017;2(3):e0023. https://www.ncbi.nlm.nih.gov/pmc/articles/PMC6133096/.
27. Meneghini R, Gibson W, Halsey D, Padgett D, Berend K, Della Valle CJ. The American association of hip and knee surgeons, hip society, knee society, and American academy of orthopaedic surgeons position statement on outpatient joint replacement. J Arthroplast. 2018;33(12):3599–601. http://www.ncbi.nlm.nih.gov/pubmed/30449455.
28. Lombardi AV, Berend KR, Adams JB. A rapid recovery program: early home and pain free. Orthopedics. 2010;33:656. http://www.slackinc.com/doi/resolver.asp?doi=10.3928/01477447-20100722-38.
29. Dowsey MM, Kilgour ML, Santamaria NM, Choong PF. Clinical pathways in hip and knee arthroplasty: a prospective randomised controlled study. Med J Aust. 1999;170(2):59–62. http://www.ncbi.nlm.nih.gov/pubmed/10026684.
30. Berger RA, Sanders SA, Thill ES, Sporer SM, Della Valle C. Newer anesthesia and rehabilitation protocols enable outpatient hip replacement in selected patients. Clin Orthop Relat Res. 2009;467(6):1424–30. http://www.ncbi.nlm.nih.gov/pubmed/19252961.
31. Carmichael NM, Katz J, Clarke H, Kennedy D, Kreder HJ, Gollish J, et al. An intensive perioperative regimen of pregabalin and celecoxib reduces pain and improves physical function scores six weeks after total hip arthroplasty: a prospective randomized controlled trial. Pain Res Manag. 2013;18(3):127–32. http://www.ncbi.nlm.nih.gov/pubmed/23748252.
32. Mears DC, Mears SC, Chelly JE, Dai F, Vulakovich KL. THA with a minimally invasive technique, multi-modal anesthesia, and home rehabilitation: factors associated with early discharge? Clin Orthop Relat Res. 2009;467(6):1412–7. http://www.ncbi.nlm.nih.gov/pubmed/19301081.
33. Sculco PK, Pagnano MW. Perioperative solutions for rapid recovery joint arthroplasty: get ahead and stay ahead. J Arthroplast. 2015;30(4):518–20. http://www.ncbi.nlm.nih.gov/pubmed/25680452.
34. Williams-Russo P, Sharrock NE, Haas SB, Insall J, Windsor RE, Laskin RS, et al. Randomized trial of epidural versus general anesthesia. Clin Orthop Relat Res. 1996;331(331):199–208. http://www.ncbi.nlm.nih.gov/pubmed/8895639.

35. Basques BA, Toy JO, Bohl DD, Golinvaux NS, Grauer JN. General compared with spinal anesthesia for total hip arthroplasty. J Bone Jt Surg. 2015;97(6):455–61. http://www.ncbi.nlm.nih.gov/pubmed/25788301.
36. Memtsoudis SG, Sun X, Chiu YL, Stundner O, Liu SS, Banerjee S, et al. Perioperative comparative effectiveness of anesthetic technique in orthopedic patients. Anesthesiology. 2013;118(5):1046–58. http://www.ncbi.nlm.nih.gov/pubmed/23612126.
37. Beaupre LA, Johnston DBC, Dieleman S, Tsui B. Impact of a preemptive multimodal analgesia plus femoral nerve blockade protocol on rehabilitation, hospital length of stay, and postoperative analgesia after primary total knee arthroplasty: a controlled clinical pilot study. Sci World J. 2012;2012:1–6. http://www.ncbi.nlm.nih.gov/pubmed/22666096.
38. Biswas A, Perlas A, Ghosh M, Chin K, Niazi A, Pandher B, et al. Relative contributions of adductor canal block and intrathecal morphine to analgesia and functional recovery after total knee arthroplasty. Reg Anesth Pain Med. 2018;43(2):1. http://www.ncbi.nlm.nih.gov/pubmed/29315129.
39. Grosso MJ, Murtaugh T, Lakra A, Brown AR, Maniker RB, Cooper HJ, et al. Adductor canal block compared with periarticular bupivacaine injection for total knee arthroplasty. J Bone Jt Surg. 2018;100(13):1141–6. http://www.ncbi.nlm.nih.gov/pubmed/29975272.
40. Sankineani SR, Reddy ARC, Eachempati KK, Jangale A, Gurava Reddy AV. Comparison of adductor canal block and IPACK block (interspace between the popliteal artery and the capsule of the posterior knee) with adductor canal block alone after total knee arthroplasty: a prospective control trial on pain and knee function in immediate postoperative period. Eur J Orthop Surg Traumatol. 2018;28(7):1391–5. http://www.ncbi.nlm.nih.gov/pubmed/29721648.
41. Lombardi AV, Berend KR, Mallory TH, Dodds KL, Adams JB. Soft tissue and intra-articular injection of bupivacaine, epinephrine, and morphine has a beneficial effect after total knee arthroplasty. Clin Orthop Relat Res. 2004;428(428):125–30. http://www.ncbi.nlm.nih.gov/pubmed/15534532.
42. Chung AS, Spangehl MJ. Peripheral nerve blocks vs periarticular injections in total knee arthroplasty. J Arthroplast. 2018;33(11):3383–8. http://www.ncbi.nlm.nih.gov/pubmed/30197218.
43. Spangehl MJ, Clarke HD, Hentz JG, Misra L, Blocher JL, Seamans DP. The Chitranjan Ranawat award: periarticular injections and femoral & sciatic blocks provide similar pain relief after TKA: a randomized clinical trial. Clin Orthop Relat Res. 2015;473(1):45–53. http://www.ncbi.nlm.nih.gov/pubmed/24706022.
44. Rosencher N, Kerkkamp HEM, Macheras G, Munuera LM, Menichella G, Barton DM, et al. Orthopedic Surgery Transfusion Hemoglobin European Overview (OSTHEO) study: blood management in elective knee and hip arthroplasty in Europe. Transfusion. 2003;43(4):459–69. http://www.ncbi.nlm.nih.gov/pubmed/12662278.
45. Hatzidakis AM, Mendlick RM, McKillip T, Reddy RL, Garvin KL. Preoperative Autologous Donation for Total Joint Arthroplasty. J Bone Jt Surg Am. 2000;82(1):89–100. http://www.ncbi.nlm.nih.gov/pubmed/10653088.
46. Alshryda S, Sarda P, Sukeik M, Nargol A, Blenkinsopp J, Mason JM. Tranexamic acid in total knee replacement. J Bone Joint Surg (Br). 2011;93-B(12):1577–85. http://www.ncbi.nlm.nih.gov/pubmed/22161917.
47. Wind TC, Barfield WR, Moskal JT. The effect of tranexamic acid on transfusion rate in primary total hip arthroplasty. J Arthroplast. 2014;29(2):387–9. http://www.ncbi.nlm.nih.gov/pubmed/23790499.
48. Duncan CM, Gillette BP, Jacob AK, Sierra RJ, Sanchez-Sotelo J, Smith HM. Venous thromboembolism and mortality associated with tranexamic acid use during total hip and knee arthroplasty. J Arthroplast. 2015;30(2):272–6. http://www.ncbi.nlm.nih.gov/pubmed/25257237.
49. Irwin A, Khan SK, Jameson SS, Tate RC, Copeland C, Reed MR. Oral versus intravenous tranexamic acid in enhanced-recovery primary total hip and knee replacement. Bone Joint J. 2013;95-B(11):1556–61. http://www.ncbi.nlm.nih.gov/pubmed/24151279.

50. Konig G, Hamlin BR, Waters JH. Topical tranexamic acid reduces blood loss and transfusion rates in total hip and total knee arthroplasty. J Arthroplast. 2013;28(9):1473–6. http://www.ncbi.nlm.nih.gov/pubmed/23886406.
51. Gilbody J, Dhotar HS, Perruccio AV, Davey JR. Topical tranexamic acid reduces transfusion rates in total hip and knee arthroplasty. J Arthroplast. 2014;29(4):681–4. http://www.ncbi.nlm.nih.gov/pubmed/24095586.
52. Anonymous. Practice guidelines for preoperative fasting and the use of pharmacologic agents to reduce the risk of pulmonary aspiration. Anesthesiology. 2017;126(3):376–93. http://insights.ovid.com/crossref?an=00000542-201703000-00014.
53. Ziemba-Davis M, Nielson M, Kraus K, Duncan N, Nayyar N, Meneghini RM. Identifiable risk factors to minimize postoperative urinary retention in modern outpatient rapid recovery total joint arthroplasty. J Arthroplast. 2019;34(7):S343–7. http://www.ncbi.nlm.nih.gov/pubmed/30956046.
54. Poehling-Monaghan KL, Kamath AF, Taunton MJ, Pagnano MW. Direct anterior versus mini-posterior tha with the same advanced perioperative protocols: surprising early clinical results. Clin Orthop Relat Res. 2015;473(2):623–31. http://www.ncbi.nlm.nih.gov/pubmed/25082624.
55. Seng BE, Berend KR, Ajluni AF, Lombardi AV. Anterior-supine minimally invasive total hip arthroplasty: defining the learning curve. Orthop Clin North Am. 2009;40(3):343–50. http://www.ncbi.nlm.nih.gov/pubmed/19576401.
56. Siddiqi A, White PB, Mistry JB, Gwam CU, Nace J, Mont MA, et al. Effect of bundled payments and health care reform as alternative payment models in total joint arthroplasty: a clinical review. J Arthroplast. 2017;32(8):2590–7. https://www.arthroplastyjournal.org/article/S0883-5403(17)30263-2/fulltext.
57. Fitzgerald SJ, Palmer TC, Kraay MJ. Improved perioperative care of elective joint replacement patients: the impact of an orthopedic perioperative hospitalist. J Arthroplast. 2018;33(8):2387–91. http://www.ncbi.nlm.nih.gov/pubmed/29691166.
58. Specht K, Kjaersgaard-Andersen P, Pedersen BD. Patient experience in fast-track hip and knee arthroplasty–a qualitative study. J Clin Nurs. 2016;25(5–6):836–45. http://www.ncbi.nlm.nih.gov/pubmed/26708610.
59. Goldstein DT, Durinka JB, Martino N, Shilling JW. Effect of preoperative hemoglobin A(1c) level on acute postoperative complications of total joint arthroplasty. Am J Orthop (Belle Mead NJ). 2013;42(10):E88–90. http://www.ncbi.nlm.nih.gov/pubmed/24278910.
60. Tait MA, Dredge C, Barnes CL. Preoperative patient education for hip and knee arthroplasty: financial benefit? J Surg Orthop Adv. 2015;24(4):246–51. http://www.ncbi.nlm.nih.gov/pubmed/26731389.
61. Lombardi AV, Viacava AJ, Berend KR. Rapid recovery protocols and minimally invasive surgery help achieve high knee flexion. Clin Orthop Relat Res. 2006;452:117–22. http://www.ncbi.nlm.nih.gov/pubmed/16957640.
62. Springer BD, Odum SM, Vegari DN, Mokris JG, Beaver WB. Impact of inpatient versus outpatient total joint arthroplasty on 30-day hospital readmission rates and unplanned episodes of care. Orthop Clin North Am. 2017;48(1):15–23. http://www.ncbi.nlm.nih.gov/pubmed/27886679.
63. Kiskaddon EM, Lee JH, Meeks BD, Barnhill SW, Froehle AW, Krishnamurthy A. Hospital discharge within 1 day after total joint arthroplasty from a veterans affairs hospital does not increase complication and readmission rates. J Arthroplast. 2018;33(5):1337–42. http://www.ncbi.nlm.nih.gov/pubmed/29275116.
64. Kolisek FR, McGrath MS, Jessup NM, Monesmith EA, Mont MA. Comparison of outpatient versus inpatient total knee arthroplasty. Clin Orthop Relat Res. 2009;467(6):1438–42. http://www.ncbi.nlm.nih.gov/pubmed/19224306.
65. Berger RA, Kusuma SK, Sanders SA, Thill ES, Sporer SM. The feasibility and perioperative complications of outpatient knee arthroplasty. Clin Orthop Relat Res. 2009;467(6):1443–9. http://www.ncbi.nlm.nih.gov/pubmed/19238499.

66. Stambough JB, Nunley RM, Curry MC, Steger-May K, Clohisy JC. Rapid recovery protocols for primary total hip arthroplasty can safely reduce length of stay without increasing readmissions. J Arthroplast. 2015;30(4):521–6. http://www.ncbi.nlm.nih.gov/pubmed/25683296.
67. Toy PC, Fournier MN, Throckmorton TW, Mihalko WM. Low rates of adverse events following ambulatory outpatient total hip arthroplasty at a free-standing surgery center. J Arthroplast. 2018;33(1):46–50. http://www.ncbi.nlm.nih.gov/pubmed/28927566.
68. Basques BA, Tetreault MW, Della Valle CJ. Same-day discharge compared with inpatient hospitalization following hip and knee arthroplasty. J Bone Jt Surg. 2017;99(23):1969–77. http://www.ncbi.nlm.nih.gov/pubmed/29206786.
69. Starks I, Wainwright TW, Lewis J, Lloyd J, Middleton RG. Older patients have the most to gain from orthopaedic enhanced recovery programmes. Age Ageing. 2014;43(5):642–8. http://www.ncbi.nlm.nih.gov/pubmed/24627354.
70. Richards M, Alyousif H, Kim JK, Poitras S, Penning J, Beaulé PE. An evaluation of the safety and effectiveness of total hip arthroplasty as an outpatient procedure: a matched-cohort analysis. J Arthroplast. 2018;33(10):3206–10. http://www.ncbi.nlm.nih.gov/pubmed/29914820.
71. Courtney PM, Froimson MI, Meneghini RM, Lee GC, Della Valle CJ. Can total knee arthroplasty be performed safely as an outpatient in the medicare population? J Arthroplast. 2018;33(7S):S28–31. http://www.ncbi.nlm.nih.gov/pubmed/29395721.
72. Nelson SJ, Webb ML, Lukasiewicz AM, Varthi AG, Samuel AM, Grauer JN. Is outpatient total hip arthroplasty safe? J Arthroplast. 2017;32(5):1439–42. http://www.ncbi.nlm.nih.gov/pubmed/28065622.
73. Parcells BW, Giacobbe D, Macknet D, Smith A, Schottenfeld M, Harwood DA, et al. Total joint arthroplasty in a stand-alone ambulatory surgical center: short-term outcomes. Orthopedics. 2016;39(4):223–8. http://www.ncbi.nlm.nih.gov/pubmed/27111079.
74. Bertin KC. Minimally invasive outpatient total hip arthroplasty. Clin Orthop Relat Res. 2005;435:154–63. http://www.ncbi.nlm.nih.gov/pubmed/15930933.
75. Lavernia CJ, Villa JM. Rapid recovery programs in arthroplasty. J Arthroplast. 2015;30(4):533–4. http://www.ncbi.nlm.nih.gov/pubmed/25680449.
76. Kelly MP, Calkins TE, Culvern C, Kogan M, Della Valle CJ. Inpatient versus outpatient hip and knee arthroplasty: which has higher patient satisfaction? J Arthroplast. 2018;33(11):3402–6. http://www.ncbi.nlm.nih.gov/pubmed/30143333.
77. DeCook CA. Outpatient joint arthroplasty: transitioning to the ambulatory surgery center. J Arthroplast. 2019;34(7):S48–50. http://www.ncbi.nlm.nih.gov/pubmed/30773355.
78. Berger RA, Jacobs JJ, Meneghini RM, Della Valle C, Paprosky W, Rosenberg AG. Rapid rehabilitation and recovery with minimally invasive total hip arthroplasty. Clin Orthop Relat Res. 2004;429(429):239–47. http://www.ncbi.nlm.nih.gov/pubmed/15577494
79. Berger RA, Sanders S, Gerlinger T, Della Valle C, Jacobs JJ, Rosenberg AG. Outpatient total knee arthroplasty with a minimally invasive technique. J Arthroplast. 2005;20(7 Suppl 3):33–8. http://www.ncbi.nlm.nih.gov/pubmed/16214000.
80. Dorr LD, Thomas DJ, Zhu J, Dastane M, Chao L, Long WT. Outpatient total hip arthroplasty. J Arthroplast. 2010;25(4):501–6. http://www.ncbi.nlm.nih.gov/pubmed/19640672.
81. Berend KR, Lombardi AV, Mallory TH. Rapid recovery protocol for peri-operative care of total hip and total knee arthroplasty patients. Surg Technol Int. 2004;13:239–47. http://www.ncbi.nlm.nih.gov/pubmed/15744696.

Chapter 19
Financial Considerations for Surgeons in the Outpatient Setting: Costs and Ownership Models

Joe Zasa

Introduction

In conjunction with the clinical and patient care aspects of an arthroplasty program, the economic reality of performing total joint arthroplasty (TJA) in an ambulatory surgery center (ASC) must also be addressed. Medicare and commercial payers see the cost benefits and the positive outcomes associated with performing total joints in ASCs. Accordingly, many surgery centers have successfully renegotiated commercial payer contracts and "carved out" the applicable arthroplasty CPT codes. However, it must be emphasized that negotiating payer contracts is only one, albeit a critical, factor when developing and growing an outpatient TJA program. There are a myriad factors inherent in establishing a successful arthroplasty program; thus, it is not as simplistic as adding yet another service line to the ASC, such as ophthalmology or endoscopy. The obvious differentiator is that high-cost implants are utilized; however, there are other factors that must be considered in order to develop a comprehensive and successful program.

In 2016, the Ambulatory Surgery Center Association (ASCA) published *Developing and Managing Surgery Centers*, the first book on ASC development and management. In that text, a methodically planned approach to developing ASCs is emphasized with a foundational business plan utilized as the "blueprint" for the project. To summarize, comprehensive planning prior to the development of an ASC begets a sound financial structure through realistic and accurate projections. This links together with the development of solid operational systems, selection of staff, administration, and anesthesia best suited for the project, and lays the groundwork for surgeon participation and sound organizational leadership committed to the best

J. Zasa (✉)
ASD Management, Dallas, TX, USA
e-mail: joezasa@asdmanagement.com

R. M. Meneghini, L. T. Buller (eds.), *Outpatient Hip and Knee Replacement*,
https://doi.org/10.1007/978-3-031-27037-6_19

interests of the ASC. Essentially, the culture of the ASC that is so critical to its long-term success begins during the planning phase.

Developing an outpatient TJA program is simply a microcosm of ASC development so, for illustrative purposes, the following highlights our process for developing an arthroplasty program and emphasizes key aspects that we believe are integral to program success.

Develop a Business Plan

A business plan is not just a proforma or financial projection; rather, it is a thorough vetting of all aspects of the arthroplasty program. Developing the business plan acts as a reference point to establish the foundation for the program.

The business plan consists of:

1. *Executive Summary*—this is a summary of the program and includes volume and financial assumptions, an explanation and support for the financial projections, the timing of the project, the surgeons involved and their level of commitment, necessary approvals, competition, projected capital expenditures, third party payer issues, expected vendor pricing particularly for implants, work and patient flow, and the overall benefits of the program.
2. *Financial Projections*—included should be:
   (a) Sources and Uses of funds showing the start-up costs for the program and how it is being funded.
   (b) Income Statement using three scenarios (low, probable, and aggressive). Two income statements should be prepared. The first is explicitly for the arthroplasty program and details revenues and direct expenses specific to the arthroplasty program. The second is an income statement for the existing ASC showing its performance before and after the joint program is implemented.
3. *Supporting Schedules*:
   (a) Existing outpatient arthroplasty volume,
   (b) Projected surgeon volume at the ASC (low, probable, and aggressive),
   (c) Revenue and payer mix assumptions,
   (d) Staffing assumptions,
   (e) Vendor implant pricing from the selected implant vendor.
   (f) Equipment requirements (tied back to the sources and uses of funds *see above*) with supporting vendor bids.
   (g) Projected construction costs from the selected contractor, if applicable, (tied back to the sources and uses of funds *see above*).

Specific Steps Required to Develop a Comprehensive Business Plan for TJA

As described above, a comprehensive plan must be developed. The following is the process we follow:

Creating and Meeting with the Implementation Team

The initial step is to identify the implementers to assist with the project. These team members with different skill sets are identified as you consider the key concepts and goals that are envisioned. A team of surgeons, anesthesiologists, nursing personnel, administrative, and business personnel is recommended. Discussing the program, its goals, and vision with a diverse group has the added benefit of establishing a "deeper dive" into the project and raises questions or issues that may have been previously overlooked. Core concepts should include patient flow, workflow, staffing requirements, preoperative and postoperative procedures, whether overnight (23 h) stay is required or envisioned, discharge protocols, equipment and construction requirements, and vendors.

Sources and Uses of Funds

What capital expenditures or start-up expenses are required? This includes new equipment and instrumentation, construction costs, and miscellaneous fees such as legal and regulatory fees.

Second, how will the capital expenditures be funded? The amount of debt or equity should be vetted. If using debt, it can be financed through equipment vendors or through local banking arrangements typically. Our experience is that vendor financing is typically slightly more expensive but does not require personal guarantees. However, construction costs must be funded by a lending institution or by using working capital reserves of the current ASC. Notwithstanding, bids should be obtained for construction costs and equipment to obtain best pricing. In sum, competition is good and shopping for equipment vendors and contractors is important. The selected bids should be scheduled in the business plan and tied back to the projections.

As a brief segue, OR room size and 23 h stay are key topics. Typically, joint surgeons are accustomed to larger operating rooms (ORs). With the standard ASC OR in the 400–450 square foot range, the typical hospital OR is in the 600–700 square foot range. While TJA can be safely performed in the standard ASC OR, the equipment and nature of the case make for tight quarters. This is not an issue for a start-up surgery center that can design larger ORs, but it is a key issue for existing centers looking to start a TJA program. Note the cost to retrofit ORs can be very expensive, so this is something that the surgeons must discuss and agree upon before significant expenditures are made. Similarly, 23-h stay must be planned from an operations standpoint (days the service is provided, dietary, and personnel) as well as from a design standpoint. Every ASC is different, but there are enhanced privacy issues when starting up a 23 h program and it will likely impact the recovery room and number of bays due to the common desire to have walls and doors in the 23 h designated area. In summary, understanding these costs are imperative in planning your program.

Initial Proforma

After understanding the start-up costs, the next step is to construct an initial projection of the economic impact of the program. Patient volume is critical so query the interested surgeons regarding how many outpatient joints they performed in the preceding 12 months and then estimate future growth. This must be a conservative estimate. We then run three scenarios using 60%, 70%, and 80% of projected volume to make conservative estimates regarding annual patient volume.

Determining expected revenue is simply a function of assessing the cases projected and assigning reimbursement from your third-party payer contracts. For Medicare, estimate based on the published rates that are being circulated for comments. If your contracts do not have reimbursement for these codes, we do not include them in this initial proforma. Once the payer mix is determined, use a weighted average of reimbursement to determine expected revenue per case.

Next, assess cost per case. You can ask for surgeon preference cards from the hospital to assess non-implant costs fairly easily. We measure supply costs and drugs and add a factor for variable expenses such as laundry, linen, transcription, and coding. For the implants, obtain vendor pricing from your device representatives.

As an example, see an initial proforma:

Total Joints Annually	300			
		60%	70%	80%
Total Cases Projected		180	210	240
Revenue per Case (avg. mix of Commercial and Medicare)		$ 13,000.00	$ 13,000.00	$ 13,000.00
Supply Cost Per Case		$ 600.00	$ 600.00	$ 600.00
Implant Cost per Case		$ 5,500.00	$ 5,500.00	$ 5,500.00
Expected Total Revenue		$ 2,340,000.00	$ 2,730,000.00	$ 3,120,000.00
Supply Costs		$ (108,000.00)	$ (126,000.00)	$ (144,000.00)
Implant Costs		$ (990,000.00)	$ (1,155,000.00)	$ (1,320,000.00)
Gross margin		$ 1,242,000.00	$ 1,449,000.00	$ 1,656,000.00

Note the term "gross margin" because the capital expenditures are not included in this and additional staffing is not included. Typically, the equipment is depreciated over 5 years, and the construction cost is depreciated depending on factors outside the scope of this chapter. Thus, for illustrative purposes, we will use the actual cash flow based on a debt model.

Gross Margin	$1,357,740	$1,584,030	$2,601,528
23 Hour Observe (30% of pts @$900/pt.	($ 162,000)	($ 189,000)	($ 216,000)
Equip/Const Loan ($500,000, 5 yrs @6%)	($ 116,000)	($116,000)	($ 116,000)
Additional Staffing	$0	$0	$0
Net Margin	$1,079,740	$1,279,030	$2,269,528

Refinement of the Projections

The initial projections provide a base for the economic impact of the project, but are simply an *initial exercise* to determine feasibility. The real key is the refinement phase. If the business plan is the meat, the "secret sauce" is this phase when developing a joint program.

There are two distinct areas of focus:

1. Implant Pricing
2. Third-Party Payer Reimbursement

The surgery center business is essentially a fixed-cost business with only one true material variable cost: medical supplies and drugs. Staffing is really more of a hybrid because the relatively small size of an ASC begets a core group of staff required whether the center does 200 cases per month or 300 cases per month. Thus, the incremental volume does not necessarily beget additional staffing. Thus, there is real economics of scale as additional volume is added as long as there is the capacity to perform the cases. For this reason, in our example above, we do not have additional staffing to accommodate the joint program and do not count staffing cost in the gross margin analysis. Each center is different and staffing is very much volume-based, so be aware of the core concept of fixed and variable costs, but staff according to your circumstances.

Compare and contrast staffing to the largest cost impacting the joint program: implant cost. The absolute best way to refine this cost is to create a RFP (request for proposal) and ask the implant vendors for their best pricing contingent upon the surgery center and surgeons using their implant on an almost exclusive basis (e.g., 90%). If the surgeons can work together and standardize implant costs, it will have a material impact on the cost of care, and hence the profitability of the program. In summary, standardize implants among the surgeons, obtain proposals from the implant vendors for best pricing tied to volume guarantees and drive your implant cost in the right direction.

As Medicare publishes its rates for TJA, third-party payers will gravitate to pricing similar to what CMS promulgates. However, this is an area where gains can be made that will be a win/win for the payers, patients, and your ASC. Note in the initial proforma (see above) we do not include volume from payers who do not pay for joint procedures in our estimates. Similarly, we do not include volume from payers who reimburse for these procedures at rates that are below the cost of the procedure. There is a real opportunity to contract with these payers and augment the proforma through additional volume by securing these contracts at favorable rates. Once you highlight that they are paying local hospitals at least two times (and typically more) than the rate you will accept for the same procedure, and stress the savings by moving this volume to your ASC, you create an opportunity for your ASC to lower the cost of care for the patient and the payer and drive volume to your ASC.

Notwithstanding, negotiating with third-party payers is more of an art than a science but it should be noted that information is key. Specifically, knowing your cost to perform the case is essential, as well as having an idea of what they are paying at your current site of service by obtaining Explanation of Benefits (EOBs) from patients or obtaining this data from databases. It must be emphasized that you have leverage if these cases are being performed at the hospital because, on average, hospitals are paid approximately two times what an ASC receives from Medicare and the third-party payers tend to follow this methodology. By showing the payer that these costly cases can be moved to a safer setting at a lower price, they are more inclined to carve out these procedures in your current contract. Additionally, by knowing your actual cost and refining the cost through vendor standardization, you have the ability to negotiate favorable rates and not undercut yourself. Remember, the first offer they make is rarely the one you will take, so shoot for 20–30% below the hospital rate and use the information to augment your contracting process.

Technology and Evolution

As a final note, as you develop a successful program be sure to highlight this progress within your community. We submit that it is important to market your arthroplasty program through social media to refine and optimize your presence on search engines and on review sites, such as Yelp. One strategy is to regularly promote patient outcomes, patient and family experiences, and cost effectiveness on your website, Facebook page, Instagram page, and in the media. A marketing expert can assist. Lastly, embrace technology. One specific example is using smartphone apps to monitor and manage pain control. These are still in their infancy but will be a key component in the delivery of care.

Conclusion

In summary, build a team of implementers to assist with your project, develop a sound and thoroughly vetted business plan that will lay the groundwork for a successful program, refine your program through implant standardization, and refined payer contracting by knowing your costs and highlighting the advantages for payers to carve out these procedures at your ASC. Finally, market and highlight the advantages of your program, patient outcomes, and savings. We are at the forefront of huge growth in TJA at ASCs. With proper and methodical planning and execution, you give your ASC the ability to be a leader in your market by developing it as a program of excellence.

Chapter 20
Outpatient Hip and Knee Arthroplasty: Implications for Hospitals, ASCs, and Payers

John R. Steele and Michael P. Bolognesi

Introduction

Hospitals, surgeons, and payers have recognized the potential benefits that outpatient total hip and total knee arthroplasty may provide for some patients. Although peer-reviewed literature on outpatient arthroplasty is evolving, multiple studies have demonstrated that outpatient total joint arthroplasty (TJA) can be safe and cost-effective compared to hospital-performed TJA in appropriately selected patients [1–6]. With this promising data and in the face of mounting cost pressures, insurers have begun covering TKA and THA performed in outpatient settings. As a result, the number of outpatient TJA surgeries has increased tremendously in recent years, with greater than one-half of primary TJA surgeries predicted to take place in the outpatient setting by 2026 [7]. The transition of large numbers of TJA surgeries to the outpatient setting will have a profound impact on hospitals, ASCs, and payers, the topic of this chapter.

In general, ASCs and payers stand to gain financially, while hospitals are likely to incur financial losses. As their market share of TJA increases, ASCs will perform more surgeries and make more money. However, TJA patients will present new challenges for them that they will have to adapt to in order to provide safe and appropriate care. Payers also stand to gain financially as they reimburse less to hospitals, surgeons, and ASCs for TJA episodes of care. Hospitals are likely to incur financial losses as they are reimbursed less for TJA episodes of care. In addition, inpatient TJA patient cohorts are likely to become sicker and costlier on average as healthier patients undergo TJA in the outpatient setting. A summary of the likely effects of growing numbers of outpatient arthroplasty on these stakeholders is summarized in Table 20.1.

J. R. Steele (✉) · M. P. Bolognesi
Department of Orthopaedic Surgery, Duke University Medical Center, Durham, NC, USA
e-mail: john.steele@duke.edu; michael.bolognesi@duke.edu

R. M. Meneghini, L. T. Buller (eds.), *Outpatient Hip and Knee Replacement*,
https://doi.org/10.1007/978-3-031-27037-6_20

Table 20.1 Summary of likely effects of outpatient arthroplasty on hospitals, ASCs, and payers

Hospitals	– Likely to incur financial losses – Inpatient TJA patient cohort likely to become sicker and costlier – Less likely to gainshare in bundled payment models
Ambulatory surgery centers	– TJA market share likely to increase, resulting in financial gains – ASCs must adapt to meet the unique challenges presented by TJA patients, including the need for increased recovery space and time, physical therapists, implant and instrument space, and sterilization equipment
Payers	– Likely to make financial gains as they reimburse surgeons and hospitals less for TJA episodes of care – Unintended, potentially deleterious consequences on bundled payment models

Implications for Hospitals

Although outpatient TJA can provide improved outcomes and cost savings in appropriately selected patients [1–6], a large proportion of TJA patients require inpatient care based on factors such as age, medical comorbidities, and socioeconomic situation. As growing numbers of younger, healthier patients undergo outpatient TJA, the risk profile of patients undergoing inpatient TJA will worsen, stressing hospitals. In addition, there is growing concern that physician and hospital/facility reimbursements for inpatient TJA will decrease as payers adjust to the lower costs of outpatient TJA [8].

CMS already reimburses differently for inpatient and outpatient surgeries, even if both are performed in the hospital. As part of the Federal Balanced Budget Act of 1997, CMS created a Medicare "outpatient prospective payment system" (OPPS) for all hospital outpatient services as an alternative to the inpatient payment system (IPPS), which reimburses hospitals for all inpatient surgery. Although these two payment systems function similarly, the facility payment for outpatient surgery is significantly lower than the hospital reimbursement for a similar inpatient procedure, due to the lower utilization of resources as well as decreased staffing and time consumption associated with outpatient care [8]. In 2018, the 50th percentile hospital reimbursement for uncomplicated TKA was approximately $11,760 under IPPS and approximately $10,123 under OPPS [9]. Similarly, prior research has shown that the average reimbursement after outpatient THA is $1155 less than inpatient THA [10]. To make matters worse, many healthcare providers and hospitals are concerned that CMS may reduce hospital reimbursements for inpatient TJA surgeries to the level of OPPS in the future.

Decreased reimbursement to hospitals for inpatient TJA would have two significant effects on hospitals. First, patients who require inpatient admission have more medical comorbidities and utilize more resources during their hospital stay, increasing the cost to the hospital associated with their admission. If reimbursement for inpatient TJA continues to decrease, hospitals may experience financial losses for their inpatient TJA patients [11]. This in turn may force hospitals to evaluate their ability to provide inpatient TJA, which would limit access to care for those patients who are not outpatient candidates.

Second, the transition of healthy patients undergoing TJA to the outpatient setting will have unintended and potentially deleterious consequences on alternative payment models including the Bundled Payments for Care Improvement (BPCI) and Comprehensive Care for Joint Replacement (CCJR) initiatives. In these payment models, participant hospitals and surgeons are financially accountable for the quality and cost of an episode of care which ranges from 30 to 90 days. Hospitals receive a single payment for the entire episode of care for a patient undergoing TJA, and are able to gainshare when the cost of admission is lower than the payment, but lose money when the cost is larger than their reimbursement. A key component of this system is that all TKA or THA patients are included so that the savings associated with healthier patients can offset the costs associated with higher resource utilization for sicker patients. If healthy TJA patients are "cherry picked" for outpatient surgery and are no longer in the alternative payment model pool, this shifts the risk profile of patients in the pool in a direction that may be costly and unsustainable for hospitals [8]. For example, one analysis of CMS data for TKA patients found that up to 40% of TKA patients leave within 24 h and could be removed from the BPCI program if they transition to outpatient, which would result in substantially less savings to hospitals of an average of $1100 per patient [12].

Implications for ASCs

As previously stated, greater than one-half of primary TJA surgeries are predicted to take place in the outpatient setting by 2026 [7]. Although some of these surgeries will occur in hospital outpatient departments (HOPDs), a large proportion will likely be performed in ASCs. As such, ASCs stand to make huge financial gains as their market share of TJAs increases. However, appropriate selection of patients that are able to undergo TJA at an ASC is essential, and ASCs will have to adapt and provide new services in order to adequately treat TJA patients' unique needs.

Multiple studies have demonstrated improved outcomes and cost savings associated with TJA performed in ASCs versus inpatient facilities or HOPDs [1–7]. However, this is predicated on appropriate patient selection, as ASCs do not offer a number of services that are important for complex patients. Whereas hospitals provide an environment where acute postoperative complications can be diagnosed and intervened upon by appropriate medical personnel, ASCs often do not. Therefore, patients with severe or multiple comorbidities are not appropriate for TJA at an ASC, and ASCs must pay special attention to indicating appropriate patients for care at their facilities. Furthermore, ASCs do not have the ability to discharge patients to acute rehabilitation facilities or skilled nursing facilities, so only patients that are unlikely to need these services are appropriately indicated to undergo TJA at an ASC.

Lastly, ASCs require emergency medical services and hospital transfer policies in place for when rare but severe complications such as vascular injury or malignant hypothermia, among others, occur [7].

There are other unique challenges to performing TJA in the ASC setting that must be considered prior to starting an outpatient TJA program at an ASC. TJA patients often take several hours to recover and must walk and practice stairs with physical therapy in order to meet discharge criteria. ASCs must therefore have physical therapy, or discharge readiness, services available and have the physical space for recovery as well as gait and stair training to occur. Next, TJA surgery requires more trays and instruments than the majority of traditional outpatient surgeries. ASCs often have less space available to house these instruments and less sterilization equipment available to sterilize instruments. This must be evaluated, and good communication between surgeons, ASCs and vendors is paramount to ensuring that appropriate equipment is available [7]. Lastly, it must be noted that the majority of ASCs are physician-owned, which may present the potential for financial conflicts of interest. In their 2018 statement on outpatient joint replacement, AAHKS recommended that "any financial conflicts related to outpatient discharge, such as ownership in an ambulatory surgery center, physician-owned distributorship or outpatient services, be transparently disclosed to the patient [13]."

Implications for Payers

Along with ASCs, payers stand to gain financially from the growth of outpatient TJA. On average, CMS reimburses hospitals less for outpatient TJA than they do for inpatient TJA. In 2018 this difference was approximately $1637 for uncomplicated TKA [9]. Thus, as the percentage of TJA surgeries performed as outpatient increases, CMS will save significant amounts of money. In addition, many surgeons and hospitals believe that CMS will decrease the reimbursement for inpatient TJA to the level of outpatient TJA, further decreasing the amount of money CMS will spend on TJA. As private payers often follow reimbursement proposed by CMS, they too will likely decrease payment to surgeons and hospitals for TJA episodes of care. Therefore, private payers will also make financial gains through decreased reimbursement for TJA.

One unintended consequence of outpatient TJA that may negatively affect CMS involves the bundled payment models which they have been implementing. As previously discussed, bundled payment models including BPCI and CCJR shift financial risk to hospitals and surgeons by paying them a fixed amount for the entire episode of care surrounding TJA. These models have been successful in terms of quality improvement and cost savings for CMS [12]. However, these models rely on having healthy patients included in the population so that the money hospitals make on these patients offsets the losses that they incur on older, sicker patients. If the younger, healthier patients are transitioned to the outpatient setting, hospitals may be at risk of losing money on performing TJA in the inpatient setting. This may in turn result in decreased hospital participation in bundled payment models and thus less cost savings overall for CMS in future payment programs [12].

Conclusion

Hospitals, surgeons, and payers have recognized the potential benefits that outpatient total hip and total knee arthroplasty can provide for appropriately selected, but not all, patients. The transition of more TJA from the inpatient to the outpatient setting will have significant effects on hospitals, ASCs, and payers. In general, ASCs stand to make financial gains as their market share of TJA increases, but TJA patients will present new challenges for them that they will have to adapt to. Payers also stand to gain financially as they reimburse less for TJA episodes of care. Hospitals are likely to incur financial losses as they are reimbursed less for TJA. In addition, they are likely to lose healthy patients to the outpatient setting, causing their inpatient TJA patient cohort to become sicker and costlier on average. This, in turn, will likely have unintended consequences on bundled payment models that may subsequently affect all of these stakeholders.

References

1. Carey K, Morgan JR, Lin MY, Kain MS, Creevy WR. Patient outcomes following total joint replacement surgery: a comparison of hospitals and ambulatory surgery centers. J Arthroplast. 2020;35(1):7.
2. Berger RA, Kusuma SK, Sanders SA, Thill ES, Sporer SM. The feasibility and perioperative complications of outpatient knee arthroplasty. Clin Orthop Relat Res. 2009;467(6):1443.
3. Huang A, Ryu JJ, Dervin G. Cost savings of outpatient versus standard inpatient total knee arthroplasty. Can J Surg. 2017;60(1):57.
4. Lovald ST, Ong KL, Malkani AL, Lau EC, Schmier JK, Kurtz SM, Manley MT. Complications, mortality, and costs for outpatient and short-stay total knee arthroplasty patients in comparison to standard-stay patients. J Arthroplast. 2014;29(3):510.
5. Shah RR, Cipparrone NE, Gordon AC, Raab DJ, Bresch JR, Shah NA. Is it safe? Outpatient total joint arthroplasty with discharge to home at a freestanding ambulatory surgical center. Arthroplasty Today. 2018;4(4):484.
6. Aynardi M, Post Z, Ong A, Orozco F, Sukin DC. Outpatient surgery as a means of cost reduction in total hip arthroplasty: a case-control study. HSS J. 2014;10(3):252.
7. DeCook CA. Outpatient joint arthroplasty: transitioning to the ambulatory surgery center. J Arthroplast. 2019;34(7s):S48.
8. Edwards PK, Milles JL, Stambough JB, Barnes CL, Mears SC. Inpatient versus outpatient total knee arthroplasty. J Knee Surg. 2019;32(8):730.
9. CMS. MLN matters MM10417 January 2018 update of the Hospital Outpatient Prospective Payment System (OPPS). 2018. https://www.cms.gov/Outreach.
10. Bertin KC. Minimally invasive outpatient total hip arthroplasty: a financial analysis. Clin Orthop Relat Res. 2005;(435):154.

11. Healy WL, Rana AJ, Iorio R. Hospital economics of primary total knee arthroplasty at a teaching hospital. Clin Orthop Relat Res. 2011;469(1):87.
12. Curtin BM, Odum SM. Unintended bundled payments for care improvement consequences after removal of total knee arthroplasty from inpatient-only list. J Arthroplast. 2019;34(7s):S121.
13. AAHKS. AAHKS statement on outpatient joint replacement. 2018. http://www.aahks.org/position-statements/outpatient-joint-replacement/.

Index

A
Acetaminophen, 38
Adductor canal block, 66
Ambulatory Surgery Center Association (ASCA), 177
Ambulatory Surgery Center Operating Room, 100
Ambulatory Surgery Center Sterile Processing, 98
Ambulatory Surgery Center Storage, 95
Ambulatory surgery centers (ASCs), 25, 94, 153, 165, 177
Ambulatory Surgical Center Quality Reporting Program (ASCQR), 159
American Academy of Orthopaedic Surgeons (AAOS), 51, 150
American Association of Hip and Knee Surgeon (AAHKS), 13, 51
American College of Cardiology/American Heart Association guidelines, 62
American College of Rheumatology (ACR), 13
American Society of Anesthesiologists, 64
American Society of Anesthesiologists Physical Status (ASA-PS) classification, 166
American Society of Regional Anesthesia, 51
Analgesics, 60
Anesthesia, 102, 152
Angiotensin-converting enzyme (ACE) inhibitors, 80
Angiotensin receptor blockers (ARB), 80
Anti-anxiety, 61
Antibiotic prophylaxis, 13
Antiemetics, 60
ASC Covered Procedures List, 85

B
Benzodiazepines, 61
Blood management, 17
  intraoperative blood management strategies, 51, 52
  preoperative optimization, 50, 51
  strategies, 105
Blood transfusions, 21
Body mass index (BMI), 10
Bundled payment model, 25, 26
Bupivacaine, 63

C
Caregiver anxiety, 138
Centers for Medicare and Medicaid Services (CMS), 1, 17, 85, 157
Charlson Comorbidity Index (CCI), 166
Chloroprocaine, 63
CMS Reporting Criteria, 161
Coagulation status, 63
Comprehensive Care for Joint Replacement (CJR) model, 157
Cooled Radiofrequency Treatment, 67
COVID-19 pandemic, 1
Cryoanalgesia, 67

R. M. Meneghini, L. T. Buller (eds.), *Outpatient Hip and Knee Replacement*, https://doi.org/10.1007/978-3-031-27037-6

D
Dexamethasone, 69
Dexamethasone's antiemetic mechanism, 60
Diagnosis-related group (DRG), 107
Discharge criteria
  anesthesia and pain management, 114, 115
  patient selection, 114
  post-discharge follow up, 118
  postoperative care and physical therapy, 117, 118
  preoperative visit, 113, 114
  surgical technique and coordination, in operating room, 116
Disease Modifying Antirheumatic Medications (DMARDS), 13
Durable medical equipment (DME), 101

E
Emergency room (ER), 135
Enhanced Recovery After Surgery (ERAS) protocols, 59
Erythropoietin supplementation, 50
Essential oils, 61
Evidence-based medicine, 127
Excellent surgical technique, 116
Executive summary, 178

F
Facia iliaca compartment blocks, 65
False negative rate, 167
False positive rate (FPR), 166
Famotidine blocks H2 receptors, 60
Femoral nerve blocks, 66
Financial projections, 178
Fluid management, 68

G
Gabanoids, 60
General anesthetic (GA) techniques, 20, 64, 152
Gross margin, 181
Group physiotherapy sessions, 130

H
High efficiency reconstructive orthopaedics, 108
Hip Disability and Osteoarthritis Outcome Score (HOOS), 123
Hospital operating room, 100
Hospital readmissions reduction program (HRRP), 161
Hospital sterile processing, 99
Hospital storage, 95
Hypotension, 80
Hypoxia, 80, 81

I
Indiana University Health Saxony Hip and Knee Center, 70
Infiltration between Popliteal Artery and Capsule of the Knee (iPACK), 67
Initial proforma, 180–181
Interoperative period
  anesthesia adjuncts for pain control, 67
  blood loss, 68
  fluid management, 68
  general anesthesia, 64
  intraoperative treatment of nausea, 69
  regional anesthesia, for hip, 64
  regional anesthesia, for knee, 65
  spinal anesthesia, 62–64
Intravenous opioid medications, 79

J
Joint replacement classes, 19

K
Ketamine drip, 67
Knee and hip arthroplasty, 160
Knee Injury and Osteoarthritis Outcome Score (KOOS), 123
Knee Society Clinical Rating Score (KSCRS), 158

L
Lateral femoral cutaneous blocks, 65
Lidocaine, 63
Lidocaine drip, 67
Liposomal bupivacaine, 67
Local infiltrative anesthesia (LIA), 65, 66

M
Malnutrition, 11
Mayo Multimodal Opioid-Sparing Pain Protocol, 39
Medical risk stratification, 70

Mepivacaine, 63
Methicillin resistant *S. aureus* (MRSA), 12
Midvastus approach, 54
Minimally invasive surgical techniques, 17, 54
Mobile-based patient engagement platforms, 123
Mobilization, 129
Modern fluid management techniques, 68
Modifiable risk factors
  antibiotic prophylaxis, 13
  diabetes, 10
  inflammatory arthropathies, 12, 13
  malnutrition, 11
  vs. non-modifiable risk factors, 9
  obesity, 10
  smoking, 11, 12
  Staphylococcus aureus screening, 12
  vitamin D, 12
Multimodal analgesia, 60
Multimodal pain control, 17
Multimodal pain management, 128, 168
Multimodal pain regimens, 105

N
Neuraxial anesthesia, 42
Non-narcotic analgesic (acetaminophen), 20
Nonsteroidal anti-inflammatory drugs (NSAIDS), 20, 60

O
Obesity, 10
Obstructive sleep apnea (OSA), 81
Ondansetron, 60, 69
Opioids, 60
Outcome assessment
  complications, 159
  healthcare costs in, 162
  patient-reported outcome measures, 158, 159
  readmissions, 160, 162
Outpatient arthroplasty, 121
Outpatient arthroplasty risk assessment (OARA) score, 18, 114, 142, 166
Outpatient total joint arthroplasty (TJA)
  anesthesia, 152
  business plan, 178
  comprehensive business plan, 179–181
  cost differences, 87
  education, 149
  hospital setting, 107, 108
  implications for ASC, 187, 188
  implications for hospitals, 186, 187
  implications for prayer, 188, 189
  in hospital setting, 109, 110
  options for staying connected, 122
  patient mindset, 85, 86
  patient selection, 147
  post-discharge physical therapy protocols, 130, 131
  prehabilitation, role of, 129
  preoperative optimization/clearing pathways, 149
  reducing institution risk, 169–171
  reducing patient risk in, 166, 167
  reducing surgeon risk, 167–169
  refinement of projections, 181, 182
  safe same-day discharge, 129
  same day discharge criteria, 87, 88, 153
  staying connected, 154
  technology and evolution, 182
  telemedicine and electronic based follow-up, 122–124
Oxford Hip Score, 158
Oxycodone, 78

P
Pain management, 158
Pain medicine, 51
Patient anxiety, 29, 30
Patient preference, 77
Patient safety, 107
Patient satisfaction, 158
Patient-reported outcome measures (PROMs), 158, 159
Perioperative hydration, 169
Perioperative period
  multimodal pain control, 60, 61
  patient optimization, 59
Peripheral nerve blocks (PNB), 42, 65
Physical therapy, 103, 117
Physical therapy discharge criteria, 129
Placebo-controlled studies, 136
Polyethylene liner exchanges, 19
Post-anesthesia care unit (PACU), 106
Post-discharge formal physical therapy, 131
Posterior capsule infiltration, 67
Postoperative Knee Society Scores, 54
Postoperative pain
  incision length and surgical technique, 53, 54
  tourniquet use, 52
  tranexamic acid, 53

Postoperative period
  nausea and vomiting, 69
  pain management, 69
  urinary retention, 70
Preoperative anemia, 50
Preoperative education, 29
Pro re nata (PRN) orders, 69
Promethazine, 60
Propofol, 81

Q
Quadratus lumborum blocks, 65

R
Randomized controlled trial, 128
Randomized total hip arthroplasty (THA), 128
Readmissions, 70, 160, 162
Regional anesthesia, 20
  for hip, 64
  for knee, 65
Regional blocks, 66
Revolutionized joint replacement surgery, 17
Routine prophylactic antibiotics, 13

S
Same-day discharge, 128
Same-day PT, 128
Scopolamine, 61
Sensory posterior articular nerves of the knee, 67
Serum fructosamine, 10
Single shot adductor canal blocks, 66
Smoking, 11, 12
Smoking cessation programs, 11
Spaced retention method, 150
Spinal anesthesia, 105
Spinal headache, 63
Staphylococcus aureus colonization, 143
Supporting schedules, 178
Surgeon anxiety, 139

T
Tachycardia, 80
Telerehabilitation, 124
TKA exposure, 54
Total hip arthroplasty (THA), 85, 97
  gabapentinoids, 40
  neuraxial anesthesia, 41, 42
  opioid receptors, 41
  periarticular injection, 43
  peripheral nerve blocks, 42
Total joint arthroplasty (TJA)
  ambulatory surgery center vs hospital, 17
  anesthesia and pain management, 20, 21
  antiemetic and anti-inflammatory effects of steroids, 40
  anxiety and patient outcomes, 136
  assessment tools for surgeons, 142
  barriers to early discharge in, 6
  caregiver anxiety, 138
  case selection, 19
  education techniques, 31, 32
  ER visits and hospital readmissions, 139, 140
  ER visits reducing, 140
  family/caregiver preparedness, 30, 31
  in free-standing ASC, 100, 101
    and hospital decontamination and sterilization areas, 99
    anesthesia, 102
    patient selection, 91, 92
    perception of space, 93–97
    physical therapy, 103
    sterile processing, 98, 100
  hospital setting, 107
  23-h observation and transfer agreements, 21
  hypotension and tachycardia, 80
  hypoxia, 80, 81
  medical evaluation and patient selection, 2, 3
    cardiac, 3
    endocrine, 4
    gastrointestinal, 4
    general medical, 3
    hematological, 3
    infectious disease, 5
    neurological/psychological, 4
    perioperative patient optimization, 5, 6
    pulmonary, 5
    renal/urology, 4
  nausea and vomiting, 81, 82
  outpatient joint replacement, 28
  pain control, 78, 79
  patient anxiety, 29, 30, 137
  patient comprehension and limitations, 30
  patient education, 19, 20, 77
  patient expectations, 28, 29
  patient selection, 18, 77
  physical therapy discharge criteria, 82
  postoperative care and follow up, 21
  preoperative education, 78

preoperative optimization, 77
reducing readmissions, 140, 141
surgeon anxiety, 139
traditional preoperative joint replacement education, 26, 27
urinary retention, 79, 80
Total knee arthroplasty (TKA), 51, 85, 97
anti-inflammatory and acetaminophen, 38
gabapentinoids, 40
neuraxial anesthesia, 41, 42
opioid receptors, 41
periarticular injection, 43
peripheral nerve blocks, 42
Tranexamic acid, 51, 53, 68
Transient neurologic symptoms, 63
Tumor necrosis factor (TNF)-alpha inhibitors, 12

U
Unicompartmental knee arthroplasty, 92
Urinary retention, 79, 80

V
VBP programs transition, 159
Vitamin and mineral supplementation, 50
Vitamin D deficiency, 12

W
Web-based protocols, 130
Western Ontario and McMaster University Osteoarthritis Index (WOMAC), 54, 158
Wound complications, 11

GPSR Compliance

The European Union's (EU) General Product Safety Regulation (GPSR) is a set of rules that requires consumer products to be safe and our obligations to ensure this.

If you have any concerns about our products, you can contact us on ProductSafety@springernature.com

In case Publisher is established outside the EU, the EU authorized representative is:

Springer Nature Customer Service Center GmbH
Europaplatz 3
69115 Heidelberg, Germany

Batch number: 08998951

Printed by Printforce, the Netherlands